Counselling Skills for Dietitians

Second Edition

Judy Gable

MSc (Nutrition), BACP Accredited Counsellor

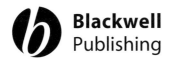
Blackwell
Publishing

© 1997, 2007 Judy Gable

Blackwell Publishing editorial offices:
Blackwell Publishing Ltd, 9600 Garsington Road, Oxford OX4 2DQ, UK
Tel: +44 (0)1865 776868
Blackwell Publishing Professional, 2121 State Avenue, Ames, Iowa 50014-8300, USA
Tel: +1 515 292 0140
Blackwell Publishing Asia Pty Ltd, 550 Swanston Street, Carlton, Victoria 3053, Australia
Tel: +61 (0)3 8359 1011

First edition published 1997
Second edition published 2007 by Blackwell Publishing Ltd

ISBN: 978 1 4051 4727 9

Library of Congress Cataloging-in-Publication Data Gable, Judy.
Counselling skills for dietitians / Judy Gable. — 2nd ed.
p. cm.
Includes bibliographical references and index.
ISBN-13: 978-1-4051-4727-9 (pbk. : alk. paper).   1. Nutrition counseling.   I. Title.
RM218.7.G33 2007
362.17′6—dc22
2006028428

A catalogue record for this title is available from the British Library

Set in 10.5/13 Plantin
By Graphicraft Limited, Hong Kong
Printed and bound in Singapore
by Markono Print Media Pte Ltd

The publisher's policy is to use permanent paper from mills that operate a sustainable forestry policy,
and which has been manufactured from pulp processed using acid-free and elementary chlorine-free
practices. Furthermore, the publisher ensures that the text paper and cover board used have met
acceptable environmental accreditation standards.

For further information on Blackwell Publishing, visit our website:
www.blackwellpublishing.com

Contents

Foreword

The concept of 'patient-centred care', which is transforming the way that health care is delivered in the UK, has always been an essential element of effective practice for dietitians. The evidence shows that advice tailored to the lifestyle of an individual, as well as their clinical condition, and based on constructive negotiation is more likely to result in positive outcomes.

The importance of effective communication is reflected in the *Standards of Proficiency* for dietitians which lay down the standards for registration by the Health Professions Council. In addition to effective and appropriate skills in relation to patient care, the *Standards* also emphasise the ability to work as a member of a multidisciplinary team. This means dietitians working together with the broad range of health professionals who are involved in the prevention and treatment of the non-communicable degenerative diseases that dominate modern health care priorities.

Counselling Skills for Dietitians is an invaluable source of insight and practical guidance, which will help those who are new to the profession to develop the skills which are so vital for effective practice. In this new edition there is also plenty for the more experienced practitioner to reflect upon. Judy Gable brings her long experience as a dietitian and a trained counsellor, together with insights gained from working with student dietitians and running in-service workshops, to produce a book of unique value. This volume will enable others to share the benefits that we have been able to enjoy at King's through Judy's involvement with the teaching of our students.

Jane Thomas
Senior Lecturer in Nutrition and Dietetics
King's College, London

Acknowledgements

I would like to thank friends and colleagues who, in giving their time and help, have contributed in so many ways to the writing of this book.

In writing the second edition I am indebted to counsellors and therapists: Peter Eastham, Janet Seller and Rodney Werninck; dietitians: Tamara Herrmann and Sue Bridgwater; and writers: Ruth Hayhurst and Jackie Kohnstamm for their feedback. In addition, I would like to thank the many dietitians who have participated in the courses that I have facilitated and the dietetic students at King's College, University of London, for their feedback which has formed so much of the material in both editions. This edition would not have materialised without the assistance I received with the first edition.

In particular, I want to thank Ashley Parnell, my co-founder and business partner at 'Voice Over' training consultancy; counsellors, psychotherapists, counselling psychologists: Jocelyn Barker, Julian Bond, Paul Hitchings; dietitians: Judith Cooke-Sanderson, Edith Elliott, Lesley Haynes, Tamara Herrmann, Dr Pat Judd, Claire O'Brien, Josette Selling; nurses, nurse-counsellors, community psychiatric nurses, social workers: Linda Beale, Kathleen Kelly, Janice Morley, Janet Powell, Jane Shackman, Angela Walton, Chris Westwell for their help with the first edition.

I would also like to thank Richard Miles at Blackwell Publishing for giving me the opportunity to write a second edition and the staff for publishing and editorial assistance. My thanks too to the following publishers: Baillière Tindall for permission to use the quote from Carl Rogers' *On Becoming a Person*; Piatkus for permission to quote from Anne Dickson's book *Difficult Conversations* and The Random House Group Ltd for permission to reprint the quote from T.A. Harris' *I'm OK, You're OK*. The guidelines for helping suicidal patients are reproduced by kind permission of Counsellors and Psychotherapists in Primary Care (CPC).

Every attempt has been made to contact copyright holders of material quoted in this book.

Introduction

When asked to write a second edition of *Counselling Skills for Dietitians* I was doubtful at first about undertaking such a task. However, once I had become involved in the project, I found myself engrossed. This process, I believe, mirrors that of many dietitians when faced with the prospect of learning counselling skills. I have heard a number of dietitians say 'Counselling skills are all very well, but I haven't the time'. In this book I hope to show how counselling skills can be integrated by dietitians so that the limited time they have with patients is utilised effectively and meaningfully for both dietitian and patient.

The first edition, published in 1997, stemmed from the needs and interest shown by dietitians who participated in the training courses in counselling skills and personal development that I facilitated during the 1990s. Many common difficulties emerged when sharing experiences about giving dietary advice to patients. For example, the patients who appeared not to heed the advice given, however clearly the dietitian thought she was putting it across, and the interviews when it became clear that the patients' difficulties were not diet related. In such situations frustration, helplessness and disenchantment frequently develop for the dietitian who then thinks 'What am I doing wrong?' or 'This patient is not worth bothering with'. Once the dietitian finds herself groaning inwardly at the prospect of seeing yet another patient, she is likely to find herself developing a routine 'spiel' to help her get through yet another busy clinic. Other difficulties arise from a lack of communication skills and a lack of self-confidence. As a result a dietitian is likely to be overly anxious, for example about giving up-to-date and accurate information or talking to certain people. This anxiety can be expressed as an inflated desire to help and to please, a fear of confrontation and a reluctance to be with someone who is emotionally distressed. A dietitian may experience such difficulties not only with patients but also with consultants, other doctors, nursing staff and managers.

This book explores ways in which these difficulties can be addressed. When writing I have drawn on my personal experience as a dietitian and a counsellor. The counselling theory in the book is based on the person-centred approach, which was originally the work of the late Carl Rogers, an eminent American psychologist, whose extensive research has moulded the development of counselling for decades. The person-centred approach, whether it is used in counselling, education or any other area, is more than a set of skills; it is both a philosophy and an attitude of mind. In the book, I focus on the use of counselling skills in clinical settings between dietitians and patients, because this is an area familiar to all dietitians. Those working in other areas and in management will find it equally useful as they discover how they can apply the skills in their communications with clinicians, colleagues and managers. The material includes exercises and clinical examples designed to stimulate self-awareness and encourage the reader to adopt a self-directed approach to learning. All examples and names given to dietitians and patients throughout the book are fictional and reference to any individual is purely accidental. I hope the reader finds the book thought provoking and satisfying to read. In my experience the material is valuable to students and so could also be useful to trainers who have an interest in interpersonal communication.

In this second edition, the basic structure of the book is unchanged. When considering what to amend and what new material to include, I realised much has progressed and much remains unchanged in the fields of both dietetics and counselling in the years since the publication of the first edition. Public awareness of counselling as an acceptable means of getting help continues to grow and counselling is increasingly widely available. Courses in counselling skills are now held in many colleges throughout the UK. Developments in the practice of health care in the past decade have placed emphasis on practitioners working in multidisciplinary teams. This means there is an even greater need for effective communication between colleagues from different disciplines if misunderstandings are to be avoided. Anxiety about roles and tasks and how these are to be performed and by whom, often leads to conflicts within teams. Meanwhile, when helping others change their eating behaviour, dietitians continue to struggle with the issue of motivation and Motivational Interviewing is a term familiar to many. Since writing the first edition there has been great interest in the use of cognitive-behavioural therapy (CBT) to help people towards changing their perceptions in the world of both counselling and dietetics. Ways in which aspects of CBT can be incorporated in patient-centred work and used for personal development are included in this edition. As the role of dietitians becomes more complex, their need for support, both professional and personal, increases. When incorporating a counsell-ing approach into their dietetic practice, dietitians need opportunities to engage in their own personal development in order to become competent practitioners. Those working interactively with patients who are emotionally vulnerable also need the support provided by the type of clinical supervision which attends to their emotional needs. In an increasingly demanding working environment, I believe it is even more necessary for dietitians to be able to maintain healthy boundaries con-cerning their role, time keeping and the extent to which they can offer confidentiality. Maintaining such boundaries supports both dietitian and patient.

As in the first edition the book is divided into four parts. Part 1 examines the counselling approach as applied to the role of the dieti-tian and distinguishes this from the dietitian as teacher or adviser. A key feature in counselling is the relationship between the helper and the person being helped. Therefore, in developing a counselling approach it is necessary for the dietitian to examine her approach and understand how this affects her relationship with her patients. Another key feature is understanding the process of change and the ways in which this can be facilitated. Exploring the ambivalence that underlies an inability to change is the basis of Motivational Interviewing, which is outlined in Chapter 4 of this edition.

Part 2 centres on the fundamental skills of listening and responding and introduces the reader to the skills of reflective responding. Used effectively, these skills further the development of the helping relation-ship. They also enable the dietitian to gain an understanding of the patient's attitude to change. In Chapter 7 I examine ways in which these skills, together with skilful questioning, can be used to make helpful interventions. The chapter now includes a section 'towards clearer thinking' which describes aspects of CBT and shows how these can be incorporated into a person-centred approach. Examples show how the skills can be used by dietitians when inviting patients to think about changing their eating behaviour.

The skills of Part 2 are applied to different settings in Part 3, which has been extensively revised in this edition. Chapter 8 describes a frame-work to use as a basis for the patient interview and introduces topics such as assessing motivation, contracting, tracking the helping process and reviewing the interview. Chapters 9–11 remain unchanged. In response to the general increased incidence of self-harm in the popula-tion, Chapter 12 contains a new section to help the dietitian cope in the event of her patient expressing suicidal thoughts. A new chapter (Chapter 13) illustrates the application of the interview framework and the counselling skills described in Parts 2 and 3. The three fictitious interviews show counselling skills being used by three dietitians in different dietetic situations.

Part 4, focusing on personal development, has been revised and expanded in this edition. In response to requests by dietitians, Chapter 14 explores ways of developing assertive behaviour and handling aggressive behaviour, not only with patients but also with colleagues in the workplace. The final chapter (Chapter 15) focuses on personal support. This includes managing stress, building self-esteem and counselling. A new section is included in this chapter which introduces the subject of mutual collegial support and describes how this can be established. Finally, the appendices have been amended and updated to include details of books for further reading and contact details of organisations associated with subjects raised in the book.

The wealth of information in the book may seem overwhelming at first. A dietitian may say 'How will I ever remember this' and 'I will forget it all when I'm with a patient'. I believe what matters most is our willingness to become better listeners more of the time, both to others and to ourselves. This involves being more skilful in the way we respond to what we hear. The skills described in Part 2 and demonstrated throughout the book are valuable life-skills. Developing, honing, polishing, and applying our listening and responding skills leads to greater understanding and opportunities for negotiation, co-operation and change. I hope this book is both useful and well used.

About the author

As a State Registered Dietitian, Judy Gable first specialised in paediatrics, where she was involved in clinical research in gastro-enterology and food sensitivity. Her MSc (Nutrition) was followed by research into diet and diabetes among the Asian community. Her interest in the psychological aspects of weight management led her to training as a counsellor. As an accredited counsellor she has worked in private practice and primary care, and has taught counselling skills to dietitians and students at King's College, University of London, for many years. She currently works in Primary Care as a counsellor in a general medical practice.

How to use this book

The following guidelines are designed to help the reader make most effective use of the book.

General points

Although chapters can be read in isolation, the reader will obtain maximum benefit by reading them in order, particularly in Part 2 where each chapter builds on the skills covered in the preceding one. References are made in each chapter to other chapters, where this is thought to reinforce the reader's learning. Each chapter contains exercises, in boxes, which are designed to increase the reader's awareness and aid learning. Dialogue is designed to demonstrate the practical application of the counselling skills and to clarify the process occurring between patient and dietitian.

Dietitians who are new to counselling

You are recommended to read Chapters 1–9, followed by Chapter 13 and Part 4. Other chapters can then be read as interest dictates.

Dietitians who work in specialised areas

You are recommended to read Chapters 1–9, followed by the relevant chapter in Part 3, followed by Chapter 13 and then Part 4. Those working in either mental health or with physical disabilities are recommended to read the introduction section of Chapter 12 in addition to the section they are interested in.

Dietitians who have completed some training in counselling skills

You are recommended to read Chapters 1, 3, 4 and 13, followed by Part 4, all of which are designed to add to your understanding. Chapter 2 and Chapters 5–9 aim to increase awareness and refresh and add to skills previously learned. The different issues raised in Parts 3 and 4 provide opportunities to clarify and develop earlier thoughts.

Notes on terminology

Dietetics is still a predominantly female profession and this fact is used in delineating gender. Dietitians are referred to as 'she' throughout and those receiving their help as 'patients'. As counselling is also a predominantly female profession, counsellors are referred to as 'she' and the person with whom they are working is referred to as a 'client'.

Names given to dietitians and patients are fictional and do not refer to individuals. Examples given are either based on my personal experiences or have been adapted so that any resemblance to specific real-life situations is purely accidental.

Part 1

A Counselling Approach

In Part 1, I introduce the reader to a counselling approach. I will be:

- exploring the role of the dietitian including her personal philosophy and qualities to develop when using a counselling approach;
- explaining some of the different approaches to counselling so that the reader can gain some background knowledge;
- considering the patient's concerns, expectations, reactions and feelings;
- exploring the nature of change and the process of adapting to it;
- focusing on the relationship between patient and dietitian and the qualities of empathy, acceptance and genuineness which the dietitian can provide;
- describing what is involved in the helping process, and how the dietitian can manage the issues of time keeping, confidentiality and referral when working with patients.

Chapter 1

The Dietitian as a Skilled Helper

'ť'is not enough to help the feeble up but to support him after'

Shakespeare: *Timon of Athens*

In this chapter I discuss:

- Teacher, adviser, guide or counsellor?
- Continuum of control
- Developing a personal philosophy
- Portrait of a dietitian using counselling skills
- Qualities of a dietitian
- Developing a counselling approach
- Different approaches to counselling

Teacher, adviser, guide or counsellor?

In a statement taken from an information leaflet produced by the British Dietetic Association (2003) the work of dietitians is described as follows:

'Dietitians are skilled in taking scientific information relating to food and health, and translating it into terms that everyone can understand.'

In other words, dietitians communicate with others on nutrition matters and dietary management. They provide a service for the sick and those who live with a chronic condition, and a service for those concerned with maintaining and promoting health. Traditionally dietitians have seen their role as that of a teacher, adviser or guide. Nowadays many describe their role as one of facilitating change or of dietary counselling. As practising dietitians know only too well, fulfilling the role is not straightforward.

Dietitians may do their best to inform, educate and facilitate using the most up-to-date knowledge at their disposal, yet patients do not always follow their information or respond to their teaching. So what goes wrong? Is it the dietitian, the patient, the diagnosis or the information given by the dietitian? Much research is done into medical diagnoses and dietetic information, and dietitians undergo lengthy training to ensure their understanding of their subject. In meeting the demands of continuing professional development they endeavour to keep abreast of current developments in the field of nutrition and dietetics.

In recent years there have also been significant developments concerned with helping people change their behaviour. The model 'Helping People Change' launched by the Health Education Authority in the 1990s helps dietitians identify the stage in a patient's process (Prochaska & DiClemente 1986). Motivational Interviewing has also been adopted by many dietitians to use within the Helping People Change model (Chapter 4). Motivational Interviewing provides a framework to help explore and resolve the ambivalence people feel about implementing change, and requires the dietitian to apply a style of interviewing that draws on characteristics of client-centred counselling (Rollnick & Miller 1995). Another form of counselling is cognitive-behavioural therapy (CBT), in which patients are introduced to strategies to help them implement change (see the section 'Different approaches to counselling' later). CBT programmes have been developed for use in the treatment of obesity (Rappoport 2000). Being able to track the change process, explore and resolve ambivalence and have strategies to show people how to implement change has greatly increased a dietitian's resources. However, patients may be willing to change and know how to do this, yet the desired outcome remains elusive. The Empowerment Model, based on principles that value the patient's right to make choices about their own health and be responsible for their own well-being, is about the helper being able to empower her patient's own resources for change (Valentine 1990; Funnell *et al.* 1991; McCann & Weinman 1996). The Helping People Change Model, motivational interviewing and the Empowerment Model have all been found to be useful in dietetic consultations with diabetic patients (Parkin 2001).

Whereas the developments described above have focused on helping obese and diabetic patients change their behaviour, dietitians working in other specialities also need resources to enable them to help their patients modify their diets. Whatever their area of work, many dietitians find the following difficult:

- dealing with a patient's reasons for not changing their eating behaviour;

- handling ambivalence when a patient is unsure about changing;
- coping with the emotions expressed by a patient;
- knowing what to say or do when a patient raises a non-dietetic problem.

In addition to her own difficulties the dietitian needs to consider those of her patients. In medical practice, research into non-compliance by patients has identified a lack of satisfaction with the consultation, a lack of understanding by the patient, and a failure by the practitioner to meet expectations, as significant factors. It was concluded that patients whose expectations are met, who are listened to, who are received in a friendly manner and are not kept waiting, experience greater satisfaction with the consultation and are more likely to comply with the practitioner's advice (Ley 1988).

It would seem that patients are more likely to be satisfied and to follow the dietitian's advice when:

- they are welcomed and seen on time;
- they feel they have been heard and understood;
- they are given information they recognise as relevant to them;
- they understand what they have to do.

It follows that, in addition to being able to give information, advice and instruction, dietitians need skills in:

- demonstrating to patients that they have been understood;
- assessing and meeting patients' needs and expectations;
- working within limited time boundaries.

How can the dietitian develop these? And the skills to employ the models described earlier? Competency in using high-level communication skills is essential if the dietitian is to be able respond to her patients' emotional needs and manage appropriately the non-dietetic problems that emerge during their work together.

Counselling skills, which offer dietitians the means to provide this quality of support for patients, have been defined for the Advice, Guidance & Counselling Lead Body as 'high level communication skills used intentionally in a manner consistent with the goals and values of counselling' (Russell, Dexter & Bond 1992).

Many health professionals use counselling skills in their work, although not all health professionals are counsellors. Those using counselling skills may also use other methods such as instructing, teaching, advising and discussing. Table 1.1 highlights the differences between these methods.

Table 1.1   Comparison of methods of communication.

Method	Purpose	Skills
Instructing	To get your message across	Ordering
Teaching	To ensure others understand the material	Explaining Demonstrating
Advising	To tell others what to do	Persuading
Discussing	To exchange points of view	Expressing oneself Listening
Counselling	To understand another To help them move towards making changes	Listening Responding helpfully

Instructing, teaching and advising centre around a one-way relationship, in which the helper is in the powerful position of being the expert in control of the situation. Discussing and counselling centre on a two-way relationship. When using counselling skills, the helper supports the person being helped to gain a sense of power and control for themselves. The nature of the relationship between the counsellor and the client, and the process which occurs within that relationship, is central to counselling. The helper who uses counselling skills develops an approach that is different from the one adopted by an instructor, teacher or adviser. This difference centres around the issue of control.

Continuum of control

The continuum of control (Eweles & Simnett 2003) relates different methods of communication to the degree of control held by the health professional, as shown in Figure 1.1. Traditionally dietitians are trained to use those methods in which they have most control. The dietitian is qualified to pass on her knowledge to others and to

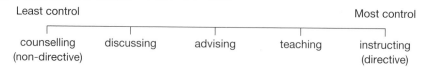

Fig. 1.1   Methods of communication related to the degree of control held by the dietitian. (Adapted from *Promoting Health – A Practical Guide to Health Education*, 5th edn, L. Eweles & I. Simnett, © (2003), with permission from Elsevier.)

provide ideas, suggestions and answers to a patient's problems with diet. She is therefore likely to be most familiar with, although not necessarily most comfortable with, methods where she has control over what takes place.

Counselling skills on the other hand require an approach in which the helper chooses to exert less control. The dietitian may feel uncomfortable with the uncertainty that this entails. However, education is of limited value when the provider has only one or two methods of delivery. The dietitian who can choose to assert her control or let go of it, depending on her purpose and the perceived needs of the patient, has a choice of approach. This enables her to be highly competent in her work.

Developing a personal philosophy

Traditionally, health professionals have been seen as experts and invested with power. This attitude is reflected in their communication with patients. Recent trends to involve patients more directly and encourage personal responsibility for health, require health professionals to examine their perception of themselves and their attitudes towards patients.

When faced with a problem, many helpers feel a responsibility to come up with a solution for the other person. Often, as the expert and the person in authority, they take this responsibility on themselves. Once the helper thinks of a solution, they see it as their job to persuade the other person to adopt and implement this.

The dietitian who thinks she should be the one to provide the solution to a problem is also likely to associate compliance by the patient with her own effectiveness. This attitude is reflected in the way in which the dietitian communicates. For example, if a patient does not follow her advice she may persuade the patient to comply in the future not only 'for their own good' but also in an attempt to feel better about herself. She is likely to use methods which allow her to be in control, such as lecturing the patient on the importance of modifying their diet or by allowing the patient to think that she also has difficulty in restraining her intake, as a way of inviting them to disclose indiscretions with their diet.

The dietitian who perceives herself as someone who knows what is best for the patient reflects a different attitude from the dietitian who thinks of herself as someone who is available to share her professional knowledge with her patients in order that they may make use of this if they choose. The latter will endeavour to provide, to the best of her ability, an environment in which a patient can feel safe, acknowledged and supported as a worthwhile human being (Chapter 3). She is likely to recognise the value of counselling skills in:

- encouraging a patient to make the choices that are best for them;
- helping a patient explore thoughts and feelings about changing their eating behaviour;
- providing a supportive relationship in which the patient feels able to make small changes for themselves.

Portrait of a dietitian using counselling skills

Sally is a dietitian who encourages her patients to take control and responsibility for themselves. She sees herself as someone whose role is to enable the patient to make their own choices. She believes that human beings are unique, that each one knows best how they feel and what they think and believe, and that although these values may not be in accord with her own, they are worthy of her respect. The respect she has for herself and others enables her to trust that her patients are able to use her information in whatever way is best for them.

In doing this she is neither naive nor irresponsible in her attitude. She is realistic and able to respond to her patients. She accepts that each individual has difficulties which are unique to them. Some of these are known to her and others are unknown. Likewise, she knows her patients are aware of some difficulties themselves and unaware of others. She sees her role as one of offering support in helping her patients understand and deal with the difficulties they have with regard to their diet (see Exercise 1.1).

Exercise 1.1

How would you describe your philosophy about helping your patients? Thinking back to the continuum of control, which methods do you feel most comfortable with?

Method	Colleagues	A patient	A group of patients
Instructing			
Teaching			
Advising			
Discussing			

Qualities of a dietitian

Dietitians frequently describe the qualities of someone who is effective in their role of helping others as someone who is:

- trustworthy;
- honest;
- reliable;
- a good listener;
- caring;
- knowledgeable;
- competent.

These are qualities which come readily to mind to most people working in the caring professions. Someone who is trustworthy and honest is thought of as someone who can be believed and relied on to do what they say they will. We trust someone and consider them honest and reliable when we experience them as being authentic, real and genuine (Rogers 2004). Genuineness (see Chapter 3) is a quality that counsellors strive continually to develop. It is demanding to be honest with oneself and to trust oneself. However, the more able we are to be this way with ourselves the more able we are to be this way with others. Openness and honesty are key characteristics of the person who is perceived to be trustworthy and reliable.

Many actions are taken which are said to be caring because they are thought to be in the best interest of another. In truth, these actions are often in the best interest of those giving the 'care', and as a result the recipient feels unheard, manipulated and disempowered. We demonstrate true caring of another when we feel empathy towards another (Chapter 3) and are willing to place ourselves at their service. We show caring by:

- giving time and attention to another;
- being fully present when listening to another;
- doing what is needed to meet the needs of another;
- helping another in their process of resolving their difficulties.

Caring is demanding yet empowering of oneself and the other person. Our ability to be available to another in this way is closely linked with our ability to establish our own boundaries, which in turn is dependent on knowing our own limits in terms of competency, and physical and emotional availability.

Developing a counselling approach

Acquiring information and monitoring competence are continual requirements for any health professional. Usually these are thought of as keeping up to date with technical and scientific developments. It is also the responsibility of the professional to develop her interpersonal and self-management skills, for without these she is unable to provide true quality care for her patients.

A dietitian who wants to develop the qualities mentioned earlier will be concerned with developing *self-awareness*. This is the key to developing genuineness and empathy (Chapter 3). Increasing self-awareness enables us to learn how we respond emotionally. This is a prerequisite if we want to help others effectively. With self-awareness we can learn to recognise our own feelings and those of another. In doing so we are less likely to attribute our own emotional response to the person to whom we are listening. In other words, we are less likely to become angry, fearful or confused by the other person and will be more able to take in what they are saying without interpreting and distorting this.

Developing self-awareness is about becoming more wholly ourselves. As Verena Tschudin (1995) succinctly says in *Counselling Skills for Nurses*: 'when we can hold the doubtful and the certain, the strong and the weak sides of ourselves in balance, then we can use ourselves positively'. She goes on to say, 'what matters is not so much that we have been "good" or "skilled helpers" but that we have been real people'.

As self-awareness grows so does 'a greater openness to and acceptance of others' (Rogers 2004). During this process we question and clarify our beliefs and experiences. These form our 'frame of reference' or the position from which we view our world. Each of us holds a different frame of reference. Using counselling skills necessitates being able to step into the frame of reference of another in order to provide empathy with someone whose experience and beliefs are different from our own. We do not have to be widowed, for example, before we can empathise with someone whose spouse has died. What is important is that we can draw on our experience of loss and suffering for the benefit of another.

Developing self-awareness is closely related to developing self-worth. An ability to value and respect oneself leads to self-acceptance and trust in oneself. As a result self-confidence grows. Patients will place greater trust in someone they sense they can rely on to be open and honest with them. Relating in this way develops a mutuality. As the dietitian's trust in herself grows, so does her willingness to trust her patients.

Imagination and intuition develop with self-trust. To be able to empathise and step into another's world requires the dietitian to use her imagination. As an ability to be empathic and genuine develops, so also does an ability to sense or intuit. Hunches provide potent material when used in an appropriate way. It is important to distinguish between hunches and assumptions, and to be aware when we are sharing a hunch, and when we are making an assumption and treating this as a fact.

An important part of building self-worth, self-value and self-respect lies in learning to care for and about oneself, in mind, body and spirit. Caring for others stems from being able to care for ourselves. If we do not feel cared for we look to others to fill our needs. Caring for the carer is therefore essential, otherwise the carer, as much as the person seeking help, is in need of receiving the care outlined earlier.

Those who are considering using a counselling approach in their work face the challenge of examining their reasons for choosing to be a member of the caring professions. Is it the hope that in providing for others they will fill their own needs? If so what are these? Is it a need for acknowledgement and recognition? Is it a desire to be thought of as 'kind' 'helpful' and 'doing something worthwhile'? A dietitian's professional practice is in question if her needs are mainly fulfilled by her patients. Yet if she has a commitment to her work and her patients is this not going to be the case? An integral part of a counsellor's training involves exploring their commitment to their own personal development. Dietitians who are thinking of using counselling skills in their work also need to explore their commitment to themselves. Part 4 outlines some aspects of personal development for the dietitian to consider.

Different approaches to counselling

Within counselling there are many different approaches based on varying beliefs about human nature. These can be broadly categorised under three headings: psychoanalytic, behavioural and humanistic.

Psychoanalytic approach

Psychodynamic counselling comes under this heading as it is based on Freud's belief that unconscious motives and drives lead us to behave in certain ways. Past experience, of which we are unaware, is relived when we encounter a similar experience in the present. Psychodynamic counselling encourages the client to explore their past in relation to the present problem. Anxiety is reduced when clients are able to make sense fully of their patterns of behaviour. The principles and practice are clearly explained by Michael Jacobs (2004) in his book *Psychodynamic Counselling in Action*. This approach is useful in health care when the patient has long-term emotional problems, suffers anxiety and talks of an unhappy childhood (Burnard 1999).

Behavioural approach

The behavioural approach is based on the belief that all behaviour is learned and so can be unlearned. The first step is to identify the undesirable behaviour and to replace this with desired behaviour by a scheme of positive reinforcement. The focus is on the behaviour and not on exploring the reasons behind the patterns of behaviour. This approach could be applied in health care with long-term behaviour problems such as those which may occur in children (Burnard 1999), and is the approach recommended by Hunt and Hilsdon (1996) in their book *Changing Eating and Exercise Behaviour*.

Cognitive approaches are frequently combined with behavioural therapies and this has led to the development of CBT, which studies have shown to be helpful for patients suffering from a range of emotional disorders including depression (Beck *et al.* 1987). CBT is based on the principle that our perception of ourselves and the world around us, that is, our point of view, shapes our thoughts (opinions, beliefs, ideas) and feelings and by learning to change our thoughts we change how we feel and behave (Beck 1989). In Chapters 7 and 15 there are examples of how aspects of CBT can be used by dietitians. The potential for CBT to be misused in a coercive way has provoked criticism (Stickley 2005). Therefore in describing how dietitians can apply the principles I have carefully considered their integration within a person-centred approach.

Humanistic approach

The aim of a humanistic approach is to 'increase the range of choices and encourage and enable the client to handle this successfully' (Rowan 1998). It is concerned with a client's thoughts, behaviour and feelings, and it is useful with problems concerning self-image and when someone believes they are powerless to change their circumstances (Burnard 1999). The humanistic approach is based on the existential philosophy that people are unique individuals essentially able to be responsible for the choices they make in their lives, rather than their actions being determined by their unconscious as in the psychodynamic approach, or learned mechanically as in the behavioural approach. In the period from 1940 to 1970, Carl Rogers formulated his theory of person-centred counselling based on his knowledge of psychoanalytic and behavioural theories, his clinical experience and a vast amount of research (Thorne 1992). A fundamental tenet of the person-centred approach is the realisation that a move towards change will occur when the qualities of empathy, acceptance and genuineness are present in a relationship (Rogers 2003).

For a more detailed exposition of the humanistic approach the dietitian is recommended to read John Rowan's (1998) account in his book *The Reality Game – a Guide to Humanistic Counselling and Therapy* and Philip Burnard's (1999) account in his book *Counselling Skills for Health Professionals*. There are many schools of therapy within each approach and many of these are concisely described in *Who Can I Talk To?* (Cooper & Lewis 1995). Many counsellors describe themselves as having an *eclectic approach* and draw on aspects from several approaches in the belief that no one approach suits every situation and that individuals benefit from the approach that most suits their needs at the time.

The *person-centred approach* forms the foundation of the counselling skills described throughout this book and is concerned with:

- enabling patients to make appropriate choices;
- helping patients express their thoughts and feelings;
- demonstrating to patients that they have been heard and understood;
- enabling patients to feel valued and respected;
- supporting patients in the actions they choose to make.

Transactional analysis, founded by Eric Berne, is another humanistic approach used in this book. Berne developed the concept of ego states calling these 'Parent, Adult and Child' (Stewart & Joines 1987). Understanding and recognising ego states can be useful as a framework for analysing an interaction when there are difficulties in communication. For example, a dietitian in Parent ego state may say to a patient, 'You shouldn't go without your breakfast.' The patient may respond from a Child ego state with, 'Well, I've never had breakfast up to now so I don't see why I should start at my age.' This conjures up an impression of a rebellious child. Alternatively, the dietitian when in Adult ego state may say, 'It is generally recognised that having some breakfast is a healthy way to start the day.' The patient who replies, 'I understand that it is healthier for me to eat something in the morning rather than start the day on an empty stomach', is then also responding from an Adult ego state.

Material is drawn from two other models where appropriate. Concepts from *family therapy* are described in Chapter 10. The aim of family therapy is to look at a family as a dynamic system and help the family members deal with their difficulties in a different way. It is not concerned with apportioning blame to an individual within the family, but rather with enabling family members to explore together the ways in which communications between them are unclear. They learn to recognise mixed messages and develop other ways of behaving towards one another. The aim of therapy is to help family members develop a different perspective on their problems and discover alternative strategies for coping.

Techniques from *neuro-linguistic programming* (NLP) developed by John Grinder, a linguist, and Richard Bandler, a mathematician and therapist (Bandler & Grinder 1979) are applied in this book where these can clarify communication. NLP includes skills such as mirroring, which can be used to great effect in creating rapport (Chapter 5). A practitioner of NLP pays great attention to detail and observation. NLP focuses on treating problems in the present without recourse to the past, and changing specific aspects of behaviour related to clearly defined problems. For example, a patient who has a phobia about heights is asked to describe in minute detail their experience of heights, including taste, smell, sight and sensation, and is then helped to change the experience by a technique called 'reframing'.

This chapter has examined the role of the dietitian and introduced some aspects of counselling. The next chapter focuses on the thoughts, feelings and behaviours associated with being a patient.

References

Bandler, R. & Grinder, J. (1979) *Frogs into Princes: Neuro Linguistic Programming*. Real People Press, Moab, USA.

Beck, A. (1989) *Cognitive Therapy and the Emotional Disorders*. International University Press, New York. Reprinted by Penguin, London (1991).

Beck, A., Rush, A.J., Shaw, B.F. & Emery, G. (1987) *Cognitive Therapy of Depression*. Guilford Press, New York.

British Dietetic Association (2003) *The Work of Registered Dietitians*. British Dietetic Association, Birmingham.

Burnard, P. (1999) *Counselling Skills for Health Professionals*, 3rd edn. Stanley Thornes Publishers, Cheltenham.

Cooper, J. & Lewis, J. (1995) *Who Can I Talk To? The User's Guide to Therapy and Counselling*. Headway Hodder & Stoughton, London.

Eweles, L. & Simnett, I. (2003) *Promoting Health – A Practical Guide*, 5th edn. Baillière Tindall, London.

Funnell, M.M., Anderson, R.M., Arnold, M.S., Barr, P.A., Donnelly, M., Johnson, P.D., Taylor-Moon, D. & White, N.H. (1991) Empowerment: an idea whose time has come in diabetes education. *Diabetes Educator.* 17, 37–41.

Hunt, P. & Hilsdon, M. (1996) *Changing Eating and Exercise Behaviour.* Blackwell Science, Oxford.

Jacobs, M. (2004) *Psychodynamic Counselling in Action,* 3rd edn. Sage Publications, London.

Ley, P. (1988) *Communicating with Patients.* Croom Helm Ltd, London.

McCann, S. & Weinman, J. (1996) Empowering the patient in the consultation: a pilot study. *Patient Education and Counseling.* 27, 227–234.

Parkin, T. (2001) An audit of the theoretical basis of education during dietetic consultations with diabetic patients. *Journal of Human Nutrition and Dietetics.* 14, 33–42.

Prochaska, J.O. & DiClemente, C.C. (1986) Towards a comprehensive model of change. In: *Treating Addictive Behaviours: Processes of Change* (eds W.R. Miller & N. Heather). Plenum, New York.

Rappoport, L. (2000) Cognitive behaviour therapy in obesity treatment. *Obesity in Practice.* 2, 13–15.

Rogers, C. (2003) *Client Centred Therapy – Its Current Practice, Implications and Theory.* Constable & Robinson, London.

Rogers, C. (2004) *On Becoming a Person.* Constable & Robinson, London.

Rollnick, S. & Miller, W.R. (1995) What is motivational interviewing? *Behavioural and Cognitive Psychotherapy.* 23, 325–334.

Rowan, J. (1998) *The Reality Game – a Guide to Humanistic Counselling and Therapy,* 2nd edn. Routledge & Kegan Paul, London.

Russell, J., Dexter, G. & Bond, T. (1992) *Differentiation Between Advice, Guidance, Befriending, Counselling Skills and Counselling.* British Association for Counselling, Rugby.

Stewart, I. & Joines, V. (1987) *TA Today – A New Introduction to Transactional Analysis.* Lifespace Publishing, Nottingham.

Stickley, T. (2005) Why is cognitive behavioural therapy so popular? *CPC Review.* 6, 5.

Thorne, B. (1992) *Carl Rogers.* Sage Publications, London.

Tschudin, V. (1995) *Counselling Skills for Nurses,* 4th edn. Baillière Tindall, London.

Valentine, V. (1990) Empowering patients for change. *Practical Diabetology.* 9, 13.

Chapter 2

The Patient

'I think it frets the saints in heaven to see
How many desolate creatures on the earth
Have learned the simple dues of fellowship
And social comfort in a hospital'

Elizabeth Barrett Browning

In this chapter I discuss:

- The patient's concerns
- The patient's feelings
- The patient's reactions
- What the patient wants
- The nature of change
- Reactions to change
- Adapting to change

The patient's concerns

The dietitian who is aware of the concerns that her patient may have is in a stronger position to provide a helping relationship (Chapter 3) than the dietitian who has not considered these. A patient who has been referred to the dietitian is likely to be concerned about what will be said and done to them and who they will be seeing. Patients are also likely to be concerned about the time involved, where the interview is to take place, how much, if anything, it is going to cost them and whether they will get satisfaction from their appointment (see Exercise 2.1). The following are some examples of questions that may occur to patients:

- Will I get there on time? Am I going to be kept waiting? How long will it take?
- Where am I going? Will I be able to find it?

- How much is the fee (if to be seen privately)? Will there be any extras?
- Will I be able to afford the diet recommended?
- Will I be weighed? Will I have to get undressed? Will I have blood taken?
- Will I be told to keep a food diary? Will I be told not to weigh myself?
- Will I understand what I am told to do? Will I be given written instructions?
- Will I have to remember everything? Will I be asked lots of questions?
- Will I be told off or criticised?
- Will the person I see be younger or older than me?
- Will they ask about my past? How much do they already know about me?

Exercise 2.1

Think of as many points as you can that may concern a patient about to see the dietitian, e.g. What will she look like?, Will she be friendly?, Will she tell me off for weighing too much/too little?

You may find it helpful to imagine or recall how you would think, feel and behave if and when you, as a patient, consult an expert, e.g. your doctor.

Their level of concern will be much related to the significance of the illness for them, in other words, what it means to them to have this condition. This may differ from the concern of the dietitian or another health professional. For example, on the one hand the dietitian may consider fluctuating blood levels a worrying sign whereas the patient may attach very little meaning to this. On the other hand the patient may be extremely concerned about the results of a particular blood test although the doctor has told them not to worry.

Patients with a **chronic** condition are likely to have concerns about:

- the abilities that they have lost, e.g. no longer able to do the job or activities they did before they became ill;
- whether life is still worth living;
- how and when they will die;
- their feelings of helplessness and dependency on others;
- what others think about them, e.g. how to cope with the social stigma attached to some conditions;

- the ways in which their condition affects their relationships and sexual activity;
- whether their needs will be met by the medical profession and/or social services.

When working with, or caring for, patients who are living with a chronic condition the dietitian or carer is likely to make the following assumptions:

- 'I've got to be kind to them and think nicely about them because they have enough to put up with.'
- 'I can't possibly understand unless I also suffer from this illness.'
- 'It's not fair to be happy myself when he/she is suffering.'

Dietitians who are aware when they themselves are making these assumptions are more likely to also be aware when other carers may be doing the same. They are better placed to:

- think about how these assumptions affect their ability to provide a helping relationship;
- empathise with those carers who may seek their help;
- recognise when patients want them to believe these assumptions, e.g. a patient may say, 'You can't possibly know what it's like for me – you haven't got what I've got.'

The patient's feelings

Feelings are powerful forces which govern our thinking and behaviour and form the foundation of our experience. Culturally, we are not encouraged to express our feelings except in times of crisis. For some people, being a patient is a crisis situation. The intensity of feeling associated with being a patient will vary from person to person depending on the situation and the patient's attitude towards it. When in hospital there is increased dependency on others and this may arouse feelings which stay near to the surface. As patients we may feel:

- afraid;
- powerless;
- vulnerable;
- bewildered and confused;
- disorientated due to disruption of the normal pattern of life;
- misunderstood;
- worried and anxious;
- ashamed;

- embarrassed;
- guilty;
- frustrated.

Our anxiety as patients may be associated with thoughts about:

- not getting the help we need;
- being rejected when we ask for help;
- our survival being under threat;
- being less of a person in some way;
- losing self-confidence and self-esteem;
- becoming dependent on others;
- being under the control of others and compelled to do something;
- the unknown;
- that the worst will happen.

A patient may find it easier to express anger than to acknowledge fear. Anger may cover disappointment, anxiety, a sense of failure, sadness and loss. It has been recognised for a long time that emotion which is bottled up and trapped within the body affects muscle tension, posture, and physical and mental well-being (Reich 1980). When we are tense we have difficulty in making decisions and are more likely to set unrealistic goals. Bottled up emotion eventually leads to the development of low self-esteem and distorted beliefs about oneself and the world in general (Burnard 1999).

Physiotherapists and remedial gymnasts are trained to recognise muscle tension. Dietitians can train themselves to observe ways in which a patient may hold tension in their body, such as pursed lips, furrowed brows and rigid shoulders. Becoming more aware of the way in which people express themselves gives the dietitian clues as to how her patient is feeling (Chapters 5 and 6).

The patient's reactions

When we are patients our health is under threat. Under conditions when we feel threatened it is normal to feel afraid and angry. 'Why me?' is a common reaction to an unwelcome change such as ill health. This question, which is often asked by newly diagnosed patients as the implications of the diagnosis sink in, is a way of expressing these emotions.

Discovering we are ill can be a *shock*. Hearing news of our diagnosis may be a tremendous blow, especially if the news is given in an inconsiderate and clumsy way. Many dietitians see patients who have come straight from their doctor, who may have had to convey some bad news. The dietitian who is able to help her patient deal with the shock is providing a truly caring service.

When we are in shock we need:

- to have someone with us;
- to be listened to;
- to have contact, e.g. a hand in ours, an arm around our shoulder.

When we come out of the shock we feel a strong *release of emotion*, often anger and fear. Dietitians who understand that this is a normal reaction and feel comfortable enough to allow someone to express their feelings are providing quality care, as the following example demonstrates.

> PATIENT: It's so hard to believe . . . the doctor says the test is positive. At first I didn't believe him. Now . . . I just want to know . . . why me . . . (*in a louder voice*) What have I done to deserve this? . . . (*begins to shout*) It's not fair . . . (*suddenly looks at dietitian*) I'm sorry . . . I shouldn't go on about it.
> DIETITIAN: (*calmly*) You have had a shock and you're angry that this is happening to you.
> PATIENT: Yes I am angry . . . and . . . (*with voice shaking*) what am I going to do? How am I going to manage? What's going to happen to me? The doctor said he'd write to my GP . . . but what can he do?
> DIETITIAN: (*calmly*) You feel scared when you think about what this means for you . . . how it will affect your life . . . and you wonder how the doctors can help you.
> PATIENT: Yes . . . (*sighs deeply*) What a mess . . . you seem to understand. It's helped being able to talk to you.

Some patients react to an unwelcome change by distancing themselves from what is happening to them. This may take the form of denying to themselves and others the significance of their illness. They make talk in a way that discounts the importance of any treatment or symptom, for example saying 'Oh I'll start my diet after my holiday' or 'The pain is nothing really – don't fuss'. They may behave as though no change has occurred and continue to live their life as though nothing has happened.

Frequently, at some stage, the patient makes a bargain with him or herself or with another person. It is as though by promising to behave in a certain way, normality will be resumed; for example, 'If I try hard with the diet for a while, maybe the diagnosis will turn out to be a mistake', or 'If I keep my appointment with the dietitian, maybe my blood tests will be normal'. Our thinking at such a time is not logical but a desperate attempt to restore our life to the way it was before the change in health occurred. Dietitians will be familiar with patients who say, 'If I do without this, can I have more of that?'. Substituting one food with another is often a practical way of managing dietary restrictions, and such a question may show understanding of the principles of substitution. On the other hand it may be an indication that a patient is having difficulty in accepting the need for dietary change.

A common reaction to a change in circumstances is to *doubt our ability to cope*. The patient who asks the dietitian 'Do you think I'll manage all right?' is expressing these doubts as much as the one who clearly says 'I don't know how I'm going to cope with this diet'. The dietitian who recognises the implied anxiety in what her patient says and responds to this demonstrates her empathy (Chapter 3). Seeking to reassure the patient with remarks such as 'You'll be all right', 'Of course you'll cope' and 'I'm sure you'll be fine', risks being perceived as patronising by the patient, who may feel diminished rather than comforted (Chapter 6). Although such reassurance seeks to allay discomfort it invites the patient to think in an unrealistic way and leads to confusion. Demonstrating empathy, however, acknowledges the reality of the patient's feelings. An empathic response is more likely to be perceived as affirming and assuring despite the discomfort.

As well as experiencing self-doubt, patients may *blame* themselves, making remarks such as 'If only I hadn't eaten so much' or 'If only I hadn't been tempted'. The underlying message is 'I'm not good enough' and 'I'm a bad person'. The dietitian is demonstrating empathy, which is invaluable in creating a helping relationship (Chapter 3), when she responds to remarks such as these by acknowledging the anger patients are expressing towards themselves. One way of doing this is to say 'I think you're being very hard on yourself' or 'You seem annoyed with yourself for eating so much'.

The patient who talks freely and openly and discloses a lot about themselves may on another occasion withdraw and be reluctant to engage in further discussion. When the dietitian is aware that this is a normal way to react, she is more able to assess the situation realistically and not blame herself unnecessarily for the lack of fruitful discussion.

Patients may distance themselves from their illness and their emotions in the following ways (see Exercise 2.2):

- Withdrawing and not talking
- Avoiding the topic by skating around it, dismissing it or diminishing it
- Being reluctant to take the necessary steps to ease the situation
- Talking about the difficulties continually without resolving them.

> **Exercise 2.2**
>
> What examples can you think of where patients behave in the ways mentioned here? Note the remarks you think they may make, e.g. 'I'm fine, the diet's no problem' (dismissing any difficulties), and how they may behave, e.g. patient pretends to be asleep (withdrawing).

What the patient wants

Many of the patient's problems are likely to be long-standing. The vulnerability of being a patient is likely to bring underlying problems and emotions to the surface. The patient may want to talk about these to someone and the dietitian may be the person they have chosen. Patients may find it easier to talk to the dietitian than the doctor because they think the dietitian has more time to listen, will be more understanding or is someone they will only see once. Some people feel more comfortable talking to someone they only see briefly, what is known as 'the stranger on the train' phenomenon (Burnard 1999).

Patients want to:

- be heard and understood;
- have the opportunity to tell their story;
- have information;
- feel able to cope;
- know they have support.

Patients know that seeing the dietitian is something to do with their diet and that some change is likely. They may know exactly what the interview entails or they may not know what to expect.

Patients may want to know:

- how important is the change in diet to their health;
- if a change in diet is a short-term measure or a lifetime change;
- if the dietitian is going to be encouraging or dismissive;
- how a change in diet is going to affect the rest of their life;
- how to manage a change in diet as well as the other changes that are happening to them.

The nature of change

Change has a ripple effect

A change in a patient's diet may lead to unforeseen changes in other areas of the patient's life. For example, it may mean changes to a whole family pattern of eating, cooking and shopping, resulting in increased anxiety and arguments within the family. The dietitian has only a limited knowledge of the patient and cannot appreciate the full meaning that the prescribed change may have for that patient. However, understanding more about the process of change can help the dietitian develop greater respect for a patient as they struggle to modify their eating behaviour.

Change occurs in a number of ways

Change may be thrust upon a patient, as when a diet is prescribed to treat an acute illness. It may be initiated by a patient, as when someone decides to modify their intake because they want to lose weight for a special occasion. It may develop over time as a result of an earlier idea, as when people gradually change their eating habits as ideas on healthy eating become more widespread.

People react and adapt to change in various ways

When a change is thrust upon us we often suffer shock and grief before we are able to come to terms with it. A person with newly diagnosed diabetes, for example, is likely to react in this way. In the struggle to adapt to enforced change we make efforts at times to reinstate the situation as it was before the change occurred. The diabetic patient who follows the newly prescribed regimen carefully for a time and then appears to give up, reflects this stage. Our reactions to change are covered more fully in the next section.

Change is paradoxical in that we both want it and do not want it

A change that we have initiated because we desire the outcome, as with the woman who goes on a diet because she wants to lose weight, seems at first to be straightforward to implement. But however much she wants the change to happen, there is likely to be a significant part of her which is anxious about the process she will have to go through to effect the change. She may also have fears about how she will be once the change has occurred. Someone who succeeds in losing excess weight will be a different shape and size. As a result of the change in her body others will relate differently to her and she will also have a different perception of herself. This may have unforeseen repercussions and give rise to a different set of problems. The patient may therefore be ambivalent about achieving the results of the change which, on the face of it, she wants to happen.

Change can have implications of which we are not aware

A modification to the diet, even though small, may have a significance for the patient that is beyond their immediate awareness. A woman who has struggled with dieting in the past will have mixed thoughts and feelings about trying another diet. Her ambivalence may reflect some underlying issues involved in changing weight. She may be unaware of these and, even if she were to become aware that these were at the root of her eating behaviour, she may not be willing to face them. She may continue to struggle with dieting and let her inner conflicts remain as they are.

Reactions to change

Reactions to change or the idea of a change are largely determined by attitude. If change is perceived as unwelcome and as a threat, we mourn the loss that the change brings. If we think of the change as welcome we respond actively. If we see it as a challenge we may rise to the occasion or feel overwhelmed and unable to cope.

We react in a characteristically ambivalent way. At first we may deny that a change is necessary. Denial may be the case even when a change has obviously taken place. For example, when someone has died the bereaved person may refuse to accept the death for some time. When we realise that a change is slowly taking place we are often reluctant to acknowledge it, as may happen when someone has a chronic wasting disease. Even when the change is one we want to initiate and know how to implement, we are often beset by misgivings: 'Am I doing the right thing?' 'Was this the best choice?'. The anxiety we feel reflects the significance we attach to the change.

We may cope with the anxiety associated with a change by talking about it with someone else. We act in the hope that 'a trouble shared is a trouble halved'. This may well produce temporary relief. In return we may receive advice (helpful or otherwise) or be diverted away from our concerns on to those of the listener who wants to talk about their own anxieties. Our confidence may be shared with others without our permission and we may regret that we have spoken. On the other hand we may find it too difficult to talk or we may not have anyone in whom we feel safe enough to confide. We may try shrugging off our anxieties, telling ourselves that things will get better in time, that there is nothing we can do about it anyway. We may distract ourselves in an attempt to assuage the discomfort by getting involved with someone or something else. We may turn to alcohol, drugs or food as a prop to help us through.

Adapting to change

Although a change may be precipitated by a single sudden event, adapting to the change takes place over time. For example, the result of a blood sugar test resulting in a diagnosis of diabetes heralds a major change in a patient's life, which takes time to accept.

Implementing change is a process made up of a series of steps in a particular direction and we make changes only to return to more familiar ways of behaving in times of stress. A patient who successfully keeps to a diet for a while returns to more established patterns of eating when feeling anxious or depressed. Any change involves giving up or letting go of something familiar and gaining something new, and the uncertainty associated with this is frightening or exciting depending upon our perception. We experience a range of emotions during change, such as hope, desire, frustration, fear, determination, confusion, hopelessness and inadequacy.

We are more likely to implement a change if we perceive that the benefits to be gained by the change outweigh those we get by continuing the existing behaviour. For example, someone who realises the benefits to their health of not smoking may decide to stop buying cigarettes. However, a smoker may not succeed in becoming a non-smoker despite taking the necessary actions to stop because they still *think of themselves* as a smoker, not a non-smoker. Similarly, a patient may understand that the risks of heart disease will be reduced if they eat less fat and know the type of foods to buy as substitutes. Despite this knowledge, they may not change their eating behaviour because it is associated with their perception of themselves as someone leading a particular way of life.

This chapter has explored the thoughts, feelings and behaviour which many experience when they are unwell. The next chapter examines the relationship between patient and dietitian.

Exercise 2.3

Make a list of changes that have occurred for you in the last year. From what you have read about the ways people react and adapt to change, reflect upon how you reacted to the changes on your list.

References

Burnard, P. (1999) *Counselling Skills for Health Professionals*, 3rd edn. Stanley Thorne Publishers Ltd, Cheltenham.

Reich, W. (1980) *Character Analysis*, 3rd edn. Simon & Schuster, New York.

Chapter 3

The Relationship Between Dietitian and Patient

'If I can provide a certain type of relationship the other person will discover within himself the capacity to use that relationship for growth and change and personal development will occur.'

Carl Rogers (2004): *On Becoming a Person*

In this chapter I discuss:

- Issues arising in the relationship between patient and dietitian
- The core conditions for a helping relationship
- Empathy
- Acceptance
- Genuineness

Issues arising in the relationship between patient and dietitian

Difficulties arise in any relationship when it is perceived as being one-sided, that is, when one person feels that the other has more *power* and that there is little they can do to influence what happens. In the relationship between patient and dietitian the dietitian is in the authoritative position as the health professional and the patient is in the less powerful position as the person seeking help. It is important for the dietitian to be aware of this imbalance. It is also important for her to recognise that her patient does have power, however limited. As well as the patient needing help from the dietitian, the dietitian also needs something from her patient, for example, their attention and co-operation. When this mutuality can be appreciated by the dietitian she is more able to foster a mutually fulfilling relationship. Her attitude

towards her patients and her perception of her role as a dietitian funda-
mentally affect her ability to develop a helping relationship.

As well as her approach, the circumstances in which the dietitian
and patient meet also affect the development of a helping relationship. The length of time they spend together and the privacy available
(Chapter 4) are just two examples. To patients it may seem that they
have little opportunity to talk freely. Similarly the dietitian may think
she has little time to listen fully.

Feelings of disillusionment, then, may develop for both patient
and dietitian with each attributing power to the other, yet neither
experiencing this for themselves. Each may have thoughts such as
'There's not much point in meeting again' and 'What am I doing this
(job) for?'. Aggressive or manipulative behaviour may be used in an
attempt to counteract the feelings of powerlessness, and may result in
blame, recrimination and a high degree of non-compliance. Patients
may vote with their feet and not keep the next appointment, and the
dietitian may heave a sigh of relief that a patient has defaulted. Clearly
when this happens a helping relationship has not been established.

There are times when patients do their best to carry out the advice
and instructions they are given. There are also times when they may
feel resentful and refuse to co-operate. Most of us can recall how we
feel when someone else tells us what we 'could' or 'should' or 'ought'
to do. As children there will have been many times when we were told
'your mother/father/teacher knows best'. We had limited experience
of the world compared with the adults who cared for us and we
needed to be told what to do and how to behave. However, when these
messages are communicated between adults they reinforce the belief
that the helper knows best. The relationship between helper and the
person being helped becomes one in which the helper continues to
be invested with the power. The person being helped is encouraged
to remain dependent on the helper for advice, and so the idea of
the professional being the powerful expert is perpetuated by health
worker and patient alike.

Dependency may be fostered when patients follow a diet because
the doctor or dietitian has said this is what they have got to do.
When this happens patients are likely to feel anxious if they do not get
the approval they want. Patient and dietitian may both see failure to
comply with dietary advice as a lack of willpower and a sign of weakness. The dietitian may then respond by trying to make the patient
feel better about themselves, or the dietitian may blame the patient as
well as herself for being ineffective.

The issues of power and dependency are manifested in transference. It is valuable for dietitians to become aware of the possibility of

transference in their relationships with patients and the ways in which this may affect their work. Transference can occur in any relationship and is a concept familiar to psychodynamic counsellors and psycho-analytic therapists. Dietitians who are interested in further reading on this subject are referred to Jacobs (2004).

As patients we are likely to feel helpless, frustrated and anxious. We may, without realising it, begin to relate to those caring for us in ways which are similar to the ways we related to parents or teachers in our childhood. When this happens transference is said to have taken place. For example, patients may feel helpless and want or expect the dietitian to solve their problem for them. They may place the dietitian in the role of a mother who is there to take care of them. The patient may say things which reflect this, such as 'What are you going to do for me then?' or 'You're going to tell me I can't eat the things I really like any more, aren't you?'. These remarks are reminiscent of a child–parent relationship. The dietitian may respond in a way which enters into this type of relationship, for example, 'It's for your own good, you know'. If she does behave in a way reminiscent of the patient's mother she is said to be in *countertransference*.

Transference is not limited to the patient. The dietitian may also project her feelings and desires onto the patient; for example, a dietitian may relate to a patient as if she were a daughter by projecting onto the patient her feelings of anxiety to do the 'right' thing and her desire for approval. Alternatively she may relate to a patient as if the patient were her child and project onto them her desire to protect or criticise.

Entering into transference and countertransference usually happens without much awareness by either party. The difficulties that arise limit the quality of help and support that the dietitian can provide. The type of relationship which develops is one in which the power is held by one person, usually the dietitian, and there is an increased dependency by the patient. The dietitian can minimise the possibility of such a relationship developing by focusing on her use of *active listening* and *reflective responding* as described in Chapters 5 and 6. In Rogers' experience, transference was less likely to build up when the helper was able to provide what he called the *core conditions* in the relationship (Rogers 2004).

The core conditions for a helping relationship

A high degree of mutual respect and a sense of self-empowerment promote a sense of equality in a relationship, with each person taking responsibility for their actions. The dietitian who wants to develop her ability to relate in this way will find the *core conditions of empathy, acceptance and genuineness* (Mearns & Thorne 1999) a rich source of material. The core conditions form the foundation of the person-centred approach and provide a relationship in which the patient feels heard, accepted and valued. As a result, the patient is more able to experiment, take risks and change behaviour. In other words the patient is more motivated to change. The dietitian too is likely to experience a greater sense of satisfaction and motivation in her work.

Empathy, acceptance and genuineness are simple words to say but they are not easy to describe, as words are a limited means of communicating an experience. Those who have received empathy and acceptance from someone who is genuine are likely to recall the experience as having been particularly meaningful. These three core conditions are so interrelated that if one is missing the others are limited. Demonstrating empathy is therefore more than a skill; it is a reflection of an underlying attitude of acceptance and honesty both towards oneself and another.

Developing an ability to provide the core conditions is demanding for the helper. It requires a high degree of self-assessment and exploration of thought patterns, feelings and behaviour, and above all a willingness to question existing beliefs and to be open to new concepts.

Empathy

It is important to distinguish empathy from sympathy. Empathy involves caring in a truly genuine and accepting way and developing a sensitive and accurate understanding of the way in which another perceives their experience, while at the same time maintaining a sense of one's own identity. When we are empathic we share another person's experience *as if* it were our own, while being aware throughout that it is not. Empathy is experienced as 'having been understood' and is empowering for the person receiving it.

When we feel sympathy we seem to take on the experience of the other person as though it were our own. We may identify with another and experience a merging with them, which can lead us to be increasingly critical or protective. Our response tends to be to criticise in the hope that the other person will see the 'error' of their ways, or to reassure in the hope that the person will feel better. However, this carries a risk of creating a barrier in the relationship (Chapter 6). The person who is receiving the sympathy may feel comforted, but on the other hand they may feel patronised and chastised.

To demonstrate empathy we need to be willing and able to gain an understanding of the world of another from their point of view. This requires us to be open and accepting of their thoughts and feelings. Empathy is about a way of *being* with another. We can demonstrate empathy through our use of active listening and reflective responding (Chapters 5 and 6) and, as we develop our ability to listen in this way, we increase our ability to be empathic. However, our ability to be empathic is limited by our own need to be heard and understood by another. Therefore the more we are able to meet our own needs the more we are able to be available to another.

As health professionals, dietitians see and hear a lot about others' pain and distress. When listening to someone in distress the dietitian may have feelings which make it difficult for her to distinguish those that belong to her and those that belong to the other person. She may feel irritable, frustrated, guilty, surprised, fearful, helpless and overwhelmed. In order to cope with this she may cut herself off emotionally or else worry greatly about the other person, which limits her ability to help effectively. It is therefore important for her to be able to understand her own reactions (Exercise 3.1).

Developing the ability to observe and acknowledge feelings appropriately is a process of personal development (see Part 4) during

---

Exercise 3.1

If possible do this exercise with a partner. Below are outlines of three 'real life' experiences of dietitians. Take each one separately. One person reads through a situation and the other listens. As you do so focus on your immediate reactions. How do you feel, what are you thinking, what action do you want to take? Discuss this with your partner.

(1) A patient you have seen once before returns for a follow-up appointment. She says, 'I've been turning a lot of things over in my mind since my last visit. I think a lot of how I feel about myself and my weight is because I was interfered with . . . as a child . . . you know . . . what do you think?'

(2) A terminally ill patient on enteral feeds says to you: 'You're very kind to take so much trouble with me. I don't know why you bother though – there's not much point is there? I'd like to die now.'

(3) A patient says, 'It's all very well for you, you're getting paid for this. You can afford to eat. Me . . . I'm unemployed with barely enough to live on and you tell me I can afford this diet. How do you know? I bet you've never known what it's like to go without.'

which the dietitian becomes more open and able to provide the core conditions.

Empathic responses

Different levels of empathy have been recognised. These range from a response which shows no understanding at all to a response in which the helper demonstrates an understanding which is beyond the client's present awareness (Mearns & Thorne 1999). In the following example four different responses are given to illustrate the various levels of empathy.

> PATIENT: I try so hard to lose weight and manage to keep to my diet most of the week. It's at weekends . . . when I'm on my own . . . I feel so lonely I just eat . . . I guess it's for comfort really.
>
> DIETITIAN 1:   (*shows no understanding*) There's no point in comfort eating – that won't help you at all.
>
> DIETITIAN 2:   (*shows partial understanding of thoughts and feelings*) That makes it really difficult for you.
>
> DIETITIAN 3:   (*shows accurate understanding of feelings and thoughts*) It's as if all the effort you've made in the week is undone at the weekends when you're on your own and feeling lonely . . . that's when you want to eat.
>
> DIETITIAN 4:   (*shows understanding beyond the patient's immediate awareness*) When you talk about being lonely and eating to comfort yourself . . . you speak very quietly . . . as though you're feeling really sad?

In the third response the dietitian reflects, by paraphrasing, what the patient has said, and in the fourth response she is focusing on the feeling which the patient is communicating through her tone of voice (Chapter 6). Empathy at a deep level involves getting a sense of what is just beyond the other person's present awareness, as in this last example. The level of empathy which is appropriate at the time depends on the relationship that the dietitian has with a particular patient. If the dietitian responds showing a depth of understanding inappropriate to the level of relationship, the patient is likely to deny what the dietitian has said and to refrain from disclosing more. Similarly, if the dietitian shows no understanding the patient is unlikely to divulge further information. By showing partial and accurate understanding, as in the second and third responses, the dietitian is indicating her acceptance and understanding of the patient.

When first practising empathic responses the dietitian may try hard to make the 'right' one. But being empathic is more than making the right response; it is about being able to sense what the other person may be thinking and feeling, and sharing this with them. The ability to do this comes with experience, increasing self-awareness, and the development of acceptance and genuineness.

Acceptance

When we attempt to understand the experience of another we show our willingness to accept them. We find it relatively easy to accept someone we like, someone we find attractive in some way, or someone who shares our beliefs and values. It is far more difficult to accept someone whose behaviour we do not understand, whose beliefs we do not share or whose attitudes we dislike. When we consider the extent of our acceptance we begin to realise just how much this is conditional upon the other person being and acting in a particular way, as the following example shows.

PATIENT: (*speaks in an accusing tone of voice*) There's no point in weighing me this week; I know I haven't lost any. I said to my husband, 'There's no point in me going to see her – she'll only tell me off'. I've no will power, that's my problem.

DIETITIAN: (*feels taken aback, thinks to herself, 'She's right – there is no point in her coming. She'll never lose any weight'. Feels hopeless, defeated. Gives a little laugh thinking she needs to be cheerful about this*) Well, we'll have to see what we can do about that won't we? Let's see what the scales have to say, shall we? (*indicates to patient to step on scales*).

PATIENT: (*without speaking steps slowly onto scales*).

The dietitian in this example finds it difficult to accept the patient when she is behaving in an aggressive manner. Her response is an attempt to get the patient to behave in the way she would like. In the following scenario the dietitian responds differently.

PATIENT: (*speaks in an accusing tone of voice*) There's no point in weighing me this week; I know I haven't lost any. I said to my husband, 'There's no point in me going to see her – she'll only tell me off'. I've no will power, that's my problem.

DIETITIAN: (*thinks 'This sounds familiar'. Recalls a recent experience while working on the computer when whatever she tried did not work as she wanted. She thought then there was no point in going on and remembers how frustrated she felt. She wonders if this is how her patient is feeling. Now feels more accepting towards her patient and wants to demonstrate her empathy*) You nearly didn't come because you were worried that if you haven't lost any weight I'd be cross with you.

PATIENT: Well aren't you?

DIETITIAN: (*gently*) No, I'm not cross with you but I'm wondering if you're feeling cross with yourself?

PATIENT: (*with a sigh*) You're right. I just can't seem to keep to the diet. Can you help me?

Acceptance involves having respect and warmth for another as a human being, regardless of who they are or what they have done. Acceptance of another relates closely to acceptance of ourselves.

There are many things we criticise about ourselves and often we do this without being fully aware of it. The more self-aware we become, the greater our self-understanding and the greater our ability to accept ourselves. The process is a painful one at times as we gain insight into the many ways in which we do not accept ourselves, the many times we put ourselves down, the difficulties we have in acknowledging our strengths, qualities and achievements, and the way in which we focus on our faults, failings and mistakes. In most cultures, we are frequently encouraged to discount our attributes, to criticise ourselves, to set ourselves high standards and demand a great deal of ourselves. Great value is placed on achievement as a source of personal satisfaction, yet there are many who despite their considerable achievements, remain extremely self-critical.

The extent to which we are critical of ourselves and critical of others limits our ability to provide acceptance. We either expect a great deal from others or underestimate them. When people do not meet our expectations we behave in various ways, for example we may persuade, manipulate and cajole them into behaving the way we want them to. If this fails we are likely to criticise them either to their face or to others or else inwardly to ourselves. As our resentment and frustration grow we may threaten, order or lecture them until we reach a point of despair, when we are likely to give up (Exercise 3.2). As shown in Chapter 6, each of these ways of responding carries a risk of creating a barrier in the relationship.

Exercise 3.2

Think of a patient you have seen recently. What are some of the things you like about them? Write these down. What are some of the things you dislike or find uncomfortable about them? Write these down. Take each item you have noted in turn and consider this in relation to yourself. For example, you may have written 'Arrived late for appointment' as one of the things you disliked.

Now think about how you keep appointments. Do you make sure you arrive early so as not to be late? Do you criticise yourself for being late? Do you blame circumstances for making you late or do you accept that you were late as a consequence of not leaving yourself enough time? What have you learned about yourself from this exercise?

The things we find unacceptable in others are those that we have difficulty in accepting within ourselves, and the qualities and characteristics we admire in others are those we admire, or would like to develop in ourselves.

Genuineness

Genuineness, which Rogers also described as congruence, means being who we truly are without front or facade (Bolton 1986), or as the philosopher Kiekegaard put it 'being that self that one truly is'. This is by no means easy. Our culture encourages us to value achievement and undervalue emotional needs, thus fostering a society which has difficulty in expressing feelings, something psychotherapist Susie Orbach (1994) describes as 'our emotional illiteracy' in her book *What's Really Going on Here?.*

The more genuine the person, the more trust we have in them. We recognise someone as genuine when what they say matches how they say it and these are both matched by their facial expression (Bandler & Grinder 1979). There is a congruence between verbal and non-verbal communication. Conversely, we recognise when there is an incongruity. In the following example the dietitian notices this.

> DIETITIAN: Hello. How are you today Mrs Jones?
> PATIENT: (*does not make eye contact but looks down at the floor. Her face is blank apart from a slight tremor of her lower lip*). I'm OK.
> DIETITIAN: (*notices incongruence between words and body language. Speaks gently*) You seem upset. Has something happened . . . do you want to tell me about it?
> PATIENT: (*begins to cry*).

Our difficulty in expressing feelings stems from childhood when we decided that certain feelings were unacceptable. We also learned that certain behaviours were unacceptable. When we are children we confuse feelings with behaviour and, as a result of our experience conclude that while we should not behave in a certain way, we should not *feel* certain feelings either. The following is an example of how the confusion can occur.

> Jane is a 3-year-old who is happy with her discovery of a bar of chocolate, which she is smearing over her face. Her mother is horrified to find her in a sticky mess. She pulls the chocolate away from Jane and smacks her, saying loudly, 'Naughty girl'. Jane starts to cry. She feels upset. She knows her mother is cross with her. In her mind she decides this means she is a bad person. Her mother picks her up and hugs her saying, 'There's no need to cry – you can have some chocolate after you've had your dinner.' Jane stops crying but feels very confused. She thinks, 'Mummy smacks me and I cry but then she hugs me and tells me not to cry.'

In order to deal with our confusion we learn to mask how we truly feel. However, if we want to help others who are in emotional distress we need to be able to recognise and acknowledge our own feelings because these are a valuable indicator, as the following example demonstrates.

> PATIENT: (*accosts dietitian in clinic waiting room, speaks in loud voice*) I was given an appointment for 10 o'clock. It's now after 11. How would you like it if you had to wait that long?
> DIETITIAN: (*speaks calmly, makes eye contact*) I wouldn't like it and would feel angry. I recognise that you are too, by the way you are pointing your finger at me.
> PATIENT: (*pauses, lowers hand*) Oh . . . sorry . . . I didn't mean to take it out on you. It's just getting to me not knowing how much longer I've got to wait.

Here the dietitian is being open and honest with the patient in acknowledging her feeling of anger and pointing out the patient's behaviour. We sense when someone is putting on a front, when there is a discrepancy between their verbal and non-verbal communication, as would be the case if the dietitian had responded as follows.

> PATIENT: (*in loud voice*) I was given an appointment for 10 o'clock. It's now after 11. How would you like it if you had to wait that long?
> DIETITIAN: (*while moving away*) Now really . . . there's no need to get into such a state. I'm sure you won't have to wait longer than is really necessary (*smiles in what she hopes is an encouraging way and walks away*).
> PATIENT: (*shakes fist at her departing back*).

As we become more open to our feelings we gradually learn that we provide empathy and acceptance when we allow ourselves to be genuine. We come to recognise that in being who we truly are, we are creating an environment in which a healthy, helping relationship can develop.

Having examined the conditions required for a helping relationship, the next chapter focuses on how the dietitian can begin to put these into practice.

References

Bandler, R. & Grinder, J. (1979) *Frogs into Princes: Neuro Linguistic Programming*. Real People Press, Moab, USA.

Bolton, R. (1986) *People Skills*. Prentice Hall, Sydney.

Jacobs, M. (2004) *Psychodynamic Counselling in Action*, 3rd edn. Sage Publications, London.

Mearns, D. & Thorne, B. (1999) *Person Centred Counselling in Action*. Sage Publications, London.

Orbach, S. (1994) *What's Really Going on Here?* Virago Press, London.

Rogers, C. (2004) *On Becoming a Person*. Constable Robinson, London.

Chapter 4

Working Together

'You keep the time you hold the space
So I feel safe and can face
Telling you what troubles me

My time with you is time for me
To think and plan what I can do
To begin to build my life anew'

Anon: To a counsellor from a client

In this chapter I discuss:

- The circumstances surrounding the dietitian's relationship with her patient
- Helping the patient
- Concerns of the dietitian
- Establishing a time boundary
- Confidentiality
- The helping process (Stages 1–3)
- Phases of change
- Helping with ambivalence
- When, how and where to refer
- How to end
- Support for the dietitian

The circumstances surrounding the dietitian's relationship with her patient

The dietitian and patient form their relationship in a variety of settings. They may meet by appointment in a clinic for an allotted time, or in a hospital setting at the request of a nurse or doctor, where the patient may either be in bed, sitting beside the bed or in a day room. They may meet in a place where there is little privacy or they may have a room to themselves. They may meet once only or on a number of occasions over an unspecified length of time. The time available may be limited to a few minutes or may last half an hour or more. The meeting may be interrupted or brought to a premature end by the dietitian's bleep, by the patient feeling unwell or by outside factors such as the arrival of visitors or the demands of medical procedures.

This variety of circumstances means the dietitian has to quickly assess what is needed and what help she can offer, while taking into account the time and privacy available. The dietitian who uses counselling skills will be concerned with creating an environment in which both she and her patient can feel relaxed and at ease together (Chapter 8). She will be helped in this by having a framework in which to fit her work (the helping process) and a model to help her understand the process of change that her patient is experiencing.

Helping the patient

Chapter 2 describes some of the concerns experienced by patients. The dietitian who appreciates these can help her patients by also taking into account the following points.

When giving the appointment

- Clarify that the patient knows where to come and at what time.
- Explain how long the appointment is for, how much the fee is and when this is to be paid (if seeing the patient privately).
- Inform the patient what the interview will be about.
- Let the patient know what the procedure will be.

At the appointment

Explain:

- how much time you have together;
- the purpose of the appointment;
- what you will be covering;
- the arrangements for future appointments (if any);
- what information you already have about the patient;
- whether the information given by the patient is confidential or to be discussed with others.

Exercise 4.1

Imagine yourself about to send an appointment to a patient. Think what you would say if you were to include each of the points mentioned. Now imagine yourself as a patient receiving the information. How would you feel and what would you think?

Exercise 4.2

Imagine yourself seeing a patient for the first time. What would you say to cover each of the points mentioned.

Concerns of the dietitian

In addition to the concerns about privacy and time described above, the dietitian is likely to be thinking about the:

- *Patients*: Will I be able to help them? If not what shall I do? Will they be friendly, approachable or rude and disagreeable?
- *Information*: Do I know enough? Is my information accurate?
- *Interview*: Will they tell me what I need to know? How can I get them to talk? How can I get them to stop talking?

The dietitian may also be asking herself how she can tell if:

- the change in diet is one that the patient wants;
- the patient thinks dietary change has been thrust upon them;
- the patient has been considering a change in diet for some time;
- dietary change is recommended by the doctor but not accepted by the patient;
- the patient has previously made attempts to change their diet.

Exercise 4.3

Close your eyes and allow yourself to relax. Now recall yourself with a patient. A specific scene may come to mind; if so, notice as much detail as you can. Be aware of how you feel. What are you thinking about the patient? It may be that your mind remains blank or that vague memories come back to you. Whatever your experience, now return yourself to the present by recalling the room in which you are sitting before slowly opening your eyes. Write down or share with a partner your experience of this exercise, in particular your thoughts and feelings.

Establishing a time boundary

Limited time is a constraint felt by many dietitians. All too often the next patient is waiting to be seen or there are other tasks waiting to be done. The dietitian hopes that the present interview will not take too long and that there will not be any interruptions. Although she knows that, theoretically, she has, say, 20 minutes for a patient, it is often difficult to keep to this in practice. Keeping to time boundaries can be seen as being strict and authoritarian. The dietitian wants to be friendly and helpful yet she realises that if she gives more time to one patient she will have less with another and may feel guilty about doing this. When this situation persists, resentment, frustration and stress can grow.

It is helpful and caring for both the patient and herself if the dietitian keeps clear time boundaries. Clarifying the time available helps the patient feel secure and safe and allows the dietitian to relax knowing that a structure has been formed. One way to do this is to explain this to the patient at the beginning of the interview.

> DIETITIAN: (*after she has introduced herself*) We have 20 minutes together this morning. If we find we want more time we can arrange another appointment before you leave.

Having established the boundaries it is important to keep to them. This is easier to do when they have been openly stated at the start. Many dietitians believe that it will take extra time if they get involved in listening to a patient's personal concerns. However, this need not be the case if the time available has been established at the start. Counsellors who listen deeply to someone's personal concerns are trained to establish clear time boundaries and to keep to these both for their own well-being and for that of their client. A dietitian will be more able to make effective use of time in a dietetic interview by stating clearly the time available and keeping to this. As a result both dietitian and patient will be more able to attend to what is being said.

Confidentiality

This is an issue at the heart of counselling because by its very nature clients are divulging personal information and sharing intimate feelings and opinions. Confidentiality is also of concern in the practice of dietetics. A statement issued by the Disciplinary Committee of the Dietitians Board (1996) makes it clear that 'dietitians must not knowingly disclose to any unauthorised person the result of investigations or any other information of a personal or confidential nature gained in the course of practice of his/her profession.'

The *Ethical Framework for Good Practice in Counselling and Psychotherapy* (British Association for Counselling and Psychotherapy 2002) states that respecting client confidentiality is a fundamental requirement for keeping trust. Those using counselling skills in medical settings may have difficulty maintaining client confidentiality, in that information about a patient needs to be shared with others concerned with the patient's care. A health professional who ensures that her patient knows the extent to which they are being offered confidentiality is providing a good standard of practice and care.

The following example shows how this code of practice can be applied in dietetic practice. In the example an interview between a patient and a dietitian is in progress. Introductions have been made and the patient is talking about her previous attempts to lose weight.

> PATIENT: (*begins to cry*) It's the same every time I try to lose weight. He has a go at me . . . he's so cruel . . . I don't know how long I can put up with it.
> DIETITIAN: (*realises the patient could disclose information of a highly personal nature and decides to make her position clear*) You seem very upset and if it would help you to talk about it to me, I'm here to listen. Whatever you say will be confidential between us although if I think, from what you tell me, that your health is in imminent risk or that anyone else may be hurt I may need to talk about this to a colleague. I would not take this step without talking to you about it first (*pauses to give patient time to consider this*). Would you like to talk to me about why you're upset?

A dietitian may find it more practical to establish confidentiality at the beginning of an interview as in the following example.

> DIETITIAN: This is the first time we've met and before we discuss your diet I want you to know that what you say to me is confidential between us. I do keep records about the dates of your appointments and your diet requirements. If I think that anything we talk about concerns your medical condition I may need to talk to my colleagues, although if this happens I would do my best to discuss this with you first.

When considering the issue of confidentiality the following questions merit discussion:

- What are the advantages to the patient and the dietitian in establishing confidentiality?
- Under what circumstances might the dietitian want to break confidentiality?

- How can the dietitian manage situations where others invite her to break confidentiality, e.g. when a doctor wants to know what she and a patient have been talking about?

Questions concerning confidentiality apply to both written and verbal communication. Dietitians are required to keep records and write in medical notes and guidance on standards for record keeping have been published jointly by the British Dietetic Association and the Dietitians Board (Eaton & Lewis 2001). These guidelines refer to the ethical aspects of keeping records and state the need to 'protect confidentiality, to ensure consent and to assist patients and clients (and their carers) to make informed decisions'. Such information may be read by many people other than those immediately concerned with the patient. In deciding what constitutes good practice the following questions, raised in a counselling context (Bond 2000), are worth consideration by dietitians.

- Who has access to the written material?
- What might this be used for?
- Why is it desirable to keep this particular information?
- How securely are records kept and for how long?

As greater computerisation of records becomes widespread, issues of access and confidentiality become more complex. Dietitians need to record clear and accurate nutritional and biochemical information in sufficient detail. The following questions concerning confidentiality between patient and dietitian also merit consideration:

- To what extent is it necessary to record information on social and personal issues in addition to nutritional and biochemical information?
- Can social and personal issues be distinguished from dietetic-related information or are they inextricably linked?
- Do patients realise their records might be read by people other than the dietitian and their doctor?
- If the dietitian does not record non-technical information but assigns this to memory, how might a subsequent interview with the patient be affected?
- If a colleague at a follow-up appointment does not have knowledge of the social and personal issues previously discussed, how might the interview with the patient be affected?
- How might a patient feel when a dietitian, having read her colleague's notes, refers to certain social or personal issues which the patient had previously talked about in confidence?
- Where does professional integrity and respect for patient confidentiality cease and professional incompetence begin?

The dietitian may find it helpful to inform her patients what she considers necessary to record, or ask them what they want or do not want her to include. The following example shows how this could be done.

> DIETITIAN: We have talked about changes in your diet and you have told me quite a lot about yourself. I have to write a record of our appointment. Is there anything you would want me to include or to leave out?
> PATIENT: Well I don't want everyone to know I've just got divorced for instance – it's none of their business. I only told you because you asked me about cooking at home and my family. I don't mind you knowing but it's nothing to do with anyone else.
> DIETITIAN: So if I note the changes you can make in your diet and that you are willing to try these out, is that all right with you? If you see another dietitian in the future you can decide then what else you want to tell her.
> PATIENT: Yes, that's fine.

The helping process

In his book *The Skilled Helper*, Egan (2004) describes three main stages in the helping process, based on providing the core conditions of empathy, acceptance and genuineness (Chapter 3). He identifies the first stage as one of helping someone to tell their story and in so doing helping them to clarify and identify their problem. The skills of active listening and building rapport are used in this stage in building a helping relationship. The second stage concerns helping someone clarify what they need and want. This may help someone to gain a different perspective, that is to develop a new way of thinking about their problem. The helper focuses on identifying patterns in feelings, thoughts and behaviour and clarifying meanings, in addition to using the skills in Stage 1. The person helped in this way feels safe enough to consider change as possible and beneficial. The third stage is concerned with developing strategies to achieve goals and includes making decisions and plans for taking action. During this stage the helper focuses on skills of problem solving and action planning.

Stage 1 – Listening to the patient's story

Although the dietitian may feel impatient and anxious to give information and advice, allowing patients time in which to tell their story is important in fulfilling *their* needs. Some patients have a greater need to talk than others and telling the story can in itself bring relief as those who know they have been fully heard are more able to clarify their problem (Egan 2004). Attending, listening and demonstrating empathy help patients tell their story and these skills are examined in detail in Chapter 5.

The skilled dietitian who, on listening to her patient, recognises the issue that is the basis of the problem, can demonstrate her empathy by reflecting this to her patient, as shown in the following example.

> PATIENT: I have to get up early to get to work on time; there's no time for breakfast. I'm lucky if I can grab a bun when I have a coffee break. If not, by lunch time I'm really hungry and sometimes there's so much to do I only have time to have a coffee at my desk.
> DIETITIAN: The problem is, how are you going to manage to have something to eat regularly with your present work schedule.
> PATIENT: Yes . . . I just can't see how I can do it . . . not every day.

Although each patient has their unique individual story, patients' problems are likely to be one or more of the following:

- How to live with their disability, e.g. diabetes?
- How to manage this in their work?
- How to live more independently?
- How to become more assertive?
- How to live with or get out of a relationship?
- How to feel more fulfilled?
- How to feel better about themselves?

Egan explains that part of the helper's task at this stage is to confront assumptions. The skill in making effective confrontations is covered in Chapter 7. In the example above the patient is saying that they 'can't see how to do it'. One way in which the dietitian can confront this is to paraphrase as follows:

> PATIENT: Yes . . . I just can't see how I can do it . . . not every day.
> DIETITIAN: There will be days when you can and days when you will find it difficult.
> PATIENT: Yes . . . that's how it is at the moment.

As the dietitian listens to the patient's story she may pick up clues about the patient's attitude towards modifying their diet. Although the patient in this example seems unable to resolve the problem of managing the diet at work, she does add 'at the moment' indicating she is not entirely closed to the idea of finding a way.

Stage 2 – Clarifying what the patient wants

A patient may not be able to express what it is they want to achieve. They may feel confused and ambivalent about this. One way to help someone clarify what they want is to ask an open question (Chapter 7) which invites the patient to consider different futures. This can be done using the phrase 'What if you were to (lose weight)?' and 'What if you did not make any changes (to your diet)?'. Continuing with open questions such as 'What do you think that would be like?' or 'What do you think might happen as a result?' invites the patient to explore the advantages and disadvantages of a particular outcome. This can help someone to clarify what is important to them. When someone can open their mind to different possibilities for the future they are more able to make choices about the actions they might take in the present, in other words to work in Stage 3.

In the following example the dietitian invites the patient to experience this more fully, using some techniques from neuro-linguistic programming (Chapter 1).

PATIENT: I can't seem to lose weight however hard I try. It's no good . . . I'm fat and I'll always be that way . . . a hopeless case.

DIETITIAN: (*invites her to consider a different future*) What would it be like for you if you were to weigh less?

PATIENT: (after long pause) I'm not sure what you mean . . . do you mean what would I look like?

DIETITIAN: (*invites her to imagine herself differently*) What would you look like? What would you be doing? How would you be feeling about yourself? What would you be thinking about yourself?

PATIENT: I'd have more energy, I'd feel lighter, brighter . . . less of an elephant.

DIETITIAN: Less of an elephant? What sort of animal would you be like?

PATIENT: I think . . . it sounds silly I know . . . but more like a giraffe . . . they're graceful and tall and slender.

The imagination is an undervalued resource in creating a future without the problem (Egan 2004). Imagery, as in the form of the elephant and the giraffe in the above example, can be powerful as a *symbol*. In the example these images are created by the patient and represent a different future *for her*. Symbols suggested by the helper are less likely to be effective.

Using the imagination to create a different future is different from using the more established form of goal setting based on rational thinking and logical argument. Goal setting needs to be realistic and specific, for example a goal to attain a certain weight. Although 'becoming a giraffe' is specific it is hardly realistic!

Patients may set goals which seem, at least on the face of it, to be attainable to them, yet to the dietitian are clearly unrealistic. This can present a difficulty for the dietitian who knows that it is not sound dietetic practice to encourage rapid weight loss, for example, but does not want to dampen the patient's motivation. In the example which follows, the patient, a woman in her mid-forties, wants to lose 12 kg (2 stone) in the month before Christmas.

> PATIENT: I really want to lose weight this time . . . everyone says I'll look much better if I lose a couple of stone . . . and I think I can . . . I'd like to for Christmas . . . it's really special this year. So what do you say . . . shall I go for it?
>
> DIETITIAN: (*reflects on what patient has said*) You're keen to lose weight before Christmas . . . (*reflects on what this seems to mean to patient*) and you'd feel better about yourself if you lost weight. (*clarifies what patient wants her to do*) You ask me what I think. (*pauses to give herself time*) I think to lose 2 stone in a month is too much to expect of yourself and not healthy to lose it so quickly. Also I think if you set yourself that goal you would become disappointed with yourself.
>
> PATIENT: You think I'm setting my sights too high?
>
> DIETITIAN: (*calmly states what she thinks*) I think if you aim for a lower target you could successfully lose some weight before Christmas and also feel you have achieved what you set out to do.

The patient is likely to feel relieved to hear this from the dietitian as she may have inwardly known she was being unrealistic yet thought she 'ought' to put herself under this pressure. She may also be unduly influenced by others who have told her that she should lose this much. By using her skills of reflective responding and stating clearly her point of view, the dietitian is demonstrating that she is taking the patient's eating behaviour seriously, which is one of the principles of good practice when working with people in eating distress (Waskett 1993).

Stage 3 – Planning ways to achieve goals

It is a significant step to move from talking about a problem to taking the necessary action which brings about change. The dietitian who phrases her questions in the form of 'How do you think you could do this?' invites the patient to consider the actions which lead towards achieving the desired goal. The patient's commitment to change is likely to be tested at this stage. It is useful to focus on small steps which are achievable as this builds up the experience of success. If we recall the paradoxical nature of change (Chapter 2), we realise there are many ways in which we can undermine our own attempts to implement change. The dietitian can help the patient become aware of likely pitfalls by asking such questions as, 'If this were to happen how could you best deal with it?'. Discussing ways and means of managing difficult situations is part of preparing to take action.

There may be times when the patient seems to be making no progress and despairs of achieving the goal. The dietitian can help by reviewing, encouraging and supporting. Below are some suggestions of how she might do this.

Reviewing

- How do you think you're managing so far?
- In what way have things improved since you began the diet?
- What do you find satisfying about the changes you have made?
- What do you find difficult?
- What would make it easier for you?

Encouraging

- When you think of what you have achieved, how do you feel?
- You have succeeded in (*name an achievement*).
- You are (*name quality*, e.g. determined, keen, motivated).

Supporting

- Does your goal still seem right for you or would you like to change it?
- In what way can I support you?
- What would help you most at the moment?
- How could you get the support you want?

By paying attention to each stage of the helping process the dietitian is demonstrating her desire to create a helping relationship with the patient (Chapter 3). She will be pacing her input to match the pace of the patient. As a result the patient will experience the interview as helpful and is more likely to feel motivated to put the desired change into practice. The dietitian, however, may feel anxious about the amount of time she is taking and think the interview should be proceeding at a faster rate than the patient seems willing to go. Understanding the phases of change described in the next section may help the dietitian to contain her frustration and increase her willingness to proceed at the patient's pace.

Phases of change

A model of change showing different phases (Prochaska & DiClemente 1986) is outlined below and fully described by Hunt and Hilsdon (1996) in Chapter 4 of their book *Changing Eating and Exercise Behaviour*. This model can be a useful framework for dietitians in assessing how ready or not a patient is to change their behaviour. Dietitians who are familiar with Prochaska and DiClemente's model will recognise the following:

- Not interested in changing
- Thinking about change
- Preparing to change
- Making changes
- Maintaining changes
- Relapsing.

Counselling skills can be used effectively to help a patient in the different phases. In the following example counselling skills are being applied in the different phases of the model.

PATIENT: The doctor sent me to see you. He said to give you this (*hands dietitian referral slip requesting dietary advice*).

DIETITIAN: (*notices patient's use of language and suspects he has come to see her because he has been told to rather than because he wants to. She reads referral*). I understand you've been having some trouble with your heart. The doctor thinks it would be useful if we discussed your diet.

PATIENT: He said I've got to go on a diet – something about having less fat.

DIETITIAN: (*notices the patient speaks as though he is following the doctor's orders, which reinforces her first impression*) The doctor thinks it would help your heart if you ate less fat. What do you think? (*raising the issue by inviting him to speak for himself*)

PATIENT: Me . . . (*gives a small shrug of his shoulders*) I don't know . . . it's not up to me is it? You're the expert, you tell me what to do.

DIETITIAN: (*noticing the patient is giving her the responsibility for changing his behaviour, states what action she can take*) I can give you some information about how to have less fat in your diet. (*gently probing*) I am wondering though if you really want to make any changes?

PATIENT: Well . . . now you mention it . . . I like my chips and roast potatoes . . . and what's a bit of meat without fat on it . . . not worth having! We've always lived to a ripe old age in my family . . . always have . . . and had good wholesome food . . . I can't see the point in changing now.

DIETITIAN: (*accepts the patient is not interested in changing, and decides to give him some information to take away and to end the interview*). Although you do not want to do anything about changing your diet at the moment, I would like to give you this leaflet to take away with you. Many people who have had heart trouble like yours have been helped by following the advice inside (*points to this in the leaflet*). You may want to read it later when you've had time to think it over (*inviting him into the next phase of the model concerned with thinking about change*).

The next example shows counselling skills being applied when a patient is already thinking about change and is preparing to make changes.

PATIENT: The doctor told me that what I eat could have something to do with what's wrong with me. I've been trying to work out what foods upset me . . . I've even written it down . . . here (*passes over notebook*) . . . look. I don't know if it's any help . . . what do you think I should do?

DIETITIAN: (*notices the frown on patient's face as she sits down on the edge of the chair and leans forward; forms impression of someone anxious 'to get it right'; decides to clarify what patient has said*) You think that changing your diet might help and you want to know what changes to make (*patient nods; decides to invite her to participate*). Shall we go through it together and see what changes you want to make?

PATIENT: (*face relaxes and shifts back into the chair*) Yes . . . that would be helpful.

The patient has now indicated that she would like some information, advice and suggestions. At a follow-up appointment, however, the patient expresses doubts about maintaining the changes discussed at her previous appointment.

PATIENT: I've been on this diet for two months now and it doesn't seem to do me any good. I don't think there's much point in going on with it.

DIETITIAN: (*notices low, flat tone of voice and difficulty in making eye contact*) You're not sure if the changes you've made have been any help.

PATIENT: At first it was worth it . . . I felt so much better for a while . . . but now . . . I'm not so sure.

DIETITIAN: (*recognises ambivalence, senses patient feels sad and helpless, invites patient to talk about this in more detail*) You've not been feeling so well lately?

PATIENT: (*eyes fill with tears, looks down at the floor*) No . . . I've had a bad week . . . everything's gone wrong.

DIETITIAN: (*realises patient may want to talk, yet aware of their limited time together*) You seem upset . . . would you like to talk about it? We've got five minutes and we can arrange to talk about your diet some other time if you want to (*giving patient the option to talk about what is troubling her or to talk about her diet*).

PATIENT: I've not told anyone yet . . . perhaps it would help to tell you.

The dietitian recognises that the most helpful action she can take is to listen. She realises that what her patient is about to say is clearly significant to the difficulty she is having in maintaining her diet. She decides this is an appropriate point to talk about confidentiality as in the example given earlier in the chapter.

Helping with ambivalence

In the example above, the dietitian recognises the ambivalence expressed by the patient when she says 'At first it was worth it. I felt so much better for a while . . . but now . . . I'm not so sure'. Such doubts may arise at any time during the process of changing one's behaviour. As in the example the dietitian who is listening closely will realise that her patient is struggling and may have lost sight of their purpose. The dietitian who is tracking the helping process will recognise that she now needs to focus on the tasks and skills of Stage 2 of the helping process described earlier in the chapter. In other words she will help her patient to clarify what they want using the skills of active listening, reflective responding and skilful questioning (Chapters 5–7). The dietitian who is familiar with 'Motivational Interviewing' will focus on giving feedback and advice and on providing a menu of options for change. Her style will be empathic and her attitude will be one of encouraging the patient to be responsible for the changes to their diet. These are key elements in Motivational Interviewing which is based on the assumption that ambivalence underlies someone's inability to change and once this has been resolved by the patient there may or may not be a need for further intervention (Rollnick & Miller 1995). Once ambivalence is resolved a patient will be able to move forward to another phase in the process of change. The guiding philosophy of Motivational Interviewing is based on client-centred counselling. However, the interpersonal style is directive and it seems that in the absence of a clear definition and with the focus on implementing techniques, Motivational Interviewing has been used in prescriptive and manipulative ways that do not accurately reflect the concept and approach (Rollnick & Miller 1995). In accordance with accepted counselling practice, the practitioner who uses Motivational Interviewing will be:

- seeking to understand another's frame of reference through active listening (Chapter 5);
- able to express acceptance and affirmation;
- eliciting and acknowledging the patient's own beliefs, thoughts and feelings about change;
- monitoring the patient's readiness to change and working with them at their pace.

If the strategies of Motivational Interviewing are used in persuasive and manipulative ways the dietitian is likely to encounter denial by the patient. As described in Chapter 2 the very nature of change is paradoxical and personal to the person making the change. Thus the dietitian cannot make the dietary alterations or lifestyle changes for the patient nor can she control the pace at which the patient deals with their ambivalence. However, she can help the patient become more aware of their thoughts, beliefs, feelings and behaviour associated with any change. If the patient and the dietitian are willing to engage in this process and the dietitian is also competent and capable of doing so, the outcome can be rewarding for both. In order to engage effectively the dietitian needs to be able to respect the patient and understand both the helping process and the different phases of the process of change. When the dietitian can sensitively apply her skills of active listening and reflective responding (Chapters 5 and 6), thereby demonstrating the 'core conditions' (Chapter 3), she may find patients willing to explore their ambivalence about changing their behaviour. When using these skills the dietitian needs to bear in mind that she is inviting a personal revelation on the part of the patient which may arouse emotional pain. An example of this occurring has been illustrated in the previous dialogue. It may also become apparent that the patient's eating behaviour is their way of coping with a deeper problem. When this is the case the dietitian may decide that any further work with the patient is outside her professional role. She will then need to consider other means of help for the patient.

When, how and where to refer

When using counselling skills the dietitian is providing in-depth support and the patient may respond by sharing problems that are outside the role of the dietitian. The nature of the problem may mean that the help needed by the patient calls for skills and competence that the dietitian does not possess. The problems caused by working beyond our limits are recognised by Sanders (2002) who states that 'in working beyond our limits we are not helping, and are probably doing damage, to the person we are trying to help as well as causing ourselves undue stress'. Exercise 4.4 will help you to define those limits.

Exercise 4.4

The following questions are designed to help you recognise and acknowledge your limits. Ask yourself:

- Do I have sufficient time to give to this patient?
- Do I have the information this patient requires?
- How confident do I feel in my ability to use counselling skills?
- What sort of problems would affect me emotionally and hinder me in my attempts to give a patient my full attention?
- Would this patient benefit from help given by someone with more knowledge and experience in this area?

Dietitians who are members of a department and part of a medical team have these resources to draw on. When discussing referral with colleagues and with patients, respect for the patient is paramount. The following guidelines, which include some taken from *First Steps in Counselling* (Sanders 2002), may be helpful:

- Invite the patient to decide what is best for themselves.
- Pass the patient on as though they were a precious gift not an awkward bundle.
- Focus on *offering* the referral to the patient not ordering.
- Make sure the patient understands that the referral is not a rejection of them but an honest attempt to help them meet their own needs.
- Make sure the patient knows that they will be welcome to seek help from the dietitian in the future.
- Make it as easy as possible for the patient to take action, e.g. give verbal and written information and directions clearly and concisely.

It is useful to have current information to hand when offering a patient information about where to go for further help. When thinking about whether a referral is appropriate or not, the counsellor or user of counselling skills will have the question, 'What do I really know about what is available locally' (Williams 1993). Compiling a local list of resources provides dietitians with contacts and information which may be useful at some stage. A list of national resources, many of whom have local branches, is given in Appendix 2.

How to end

The end of a relationship with a patient is as important as the beginning. When a patient is seen for a one-off consultation the ending process takes place in the same session as the beginning process and, of necessity, both will be brief. When the dietitian and patient have met several times the last meeting is clearly a time to attend to the ending of their work together. Many of us have had painful experiences of endings which feel like a severance or a death. The thought of another ending can arouse anxiety for many people, particularly when a patient or dietitian have formed a strong attachment. This may be the case if the patient's illness has been life-threatening or if their relationship has become established over a long period of time.

People deal with endings in various ways. Some avoid the last meeting by not turning up or cancelling the appointment, often at the last minute. Others may not want to leave and procrastinate by introducing other topics or asking further questions. Most dietitians will be familiar with the situation where the patient asks a significant question as the appointment is drawing to a close. Some patients announce a change or give an important piece of information as they are going out of the door. When this happens the dietitian may feel surprised initially and then frustrated. However, the patient may have been biding their time and 'testing the waters', only feeling safe enough to risk making the remark on leaving. By acknowledging apparently 'throwaway' remarks rather than letting them go without comment, the dietitian demonstrates she has heard. Rather than extending the appointment and getting behind with subsequent ones, the dietitian could offer the patient another appointment, thereby giving the patient an opportunity to raise the subject again if they wish. This demonstrates respect for the patient while maintaining a clear working arrangement for both dietitian and patient.

A planned ending provides an opportunity for the patient and the dietitian to part with a sense that their work together is complete. When the sense of completion is absent both people can be left with feelings of dissatisfaction. The following points are worth considering when planning a final session with a patient:

- Allow time to review as previously described.
- Invite questions, e.g. 'is there anything else you would like to ask me?'.
- Give information about further support as appropriate, e.g. the telephone number of the dietetic department.
- Share with the patient your observations on their progress in the time you have known them.
- Share your experience of working with them, e.g.:

  'I have enjoyed working with you.'
  'We have sorted out some problems together.'
  'We don't seem to have made much headway.'
  'I don't think either of us found it easy yet we seem to have sorted out a few things.'

Support for the dietitian

When saying goodbye to a patient a dietitian may feel:

- relief that she is no longer working with this person;
- sadness that the relationship has come to an end;
- pleasure that the patient is able to manage without help;

- satisfaction that she has done a good job;
- anxiety about how the patient will cope;
- concern that she could have done more;
- frustration about the unsatisfactory way things turned out;
- annoyed with herself and guilty that she made mistakes.

A particular relationship may bring to the surface a variety of issues for the dietitian to deal with. Having personal support and someone with whom to talk these through in a safe environment is important if a helper is to provide quality help for others. For this reason counsellors are required by the ethical framework of their professional body, the British Association for Counselling and Psychotherapy, to be in regular and ongoing counselling supervision, which is independent of any managerial relationship. This framework is also applicable to users of counselling skills (British Association for Counselling and Psychotherapy 2002).

Supervision is about taking an overview, in the presence of someone with experience, 'at what you and your patient have said and done and is a central task so that you are better informed and empowered to practise' (Houston 1995). The relationship between supervisor and the person supervised, where both have a high commitment to understanding and learning, is a key issue in fulfilling this aim (Shohet & Wilmot 1991). Dietitians who use counselling skills are advised to consider how they can get similar support for themselves.

This chapter highlights the way in which the dietitian can create a working environment in which counselling skills can be effectively used. The issues raised are further explored and applied in the patient interview in Part 3 of this book. Firstly though it is necessary to examine and develop the counselling skills of active listening and reflective responding.

References

Bond, T. (2000) *Standards and Ethics for Counselling in Action*. Sage Publications, London.

British Association for Counselling and Psychotherapy (2002) *Ethical Framework for Good Practice in Counselling and Psychotherapy*. British Association for Counselling and Psychotherapy, Rugby.

Disciplinary Committee of the Dietitians Board (1996) *Statement of Conduct*. Council for Professions Supplementary to Medicine, London.

Eaton, J. & Lewis, B. (2001) *Guidance on Standards for Records and Record Keeping*, 2nd edn. British Dietetic Association, Birmingham and Dietitians Board, London.

Egan, G. (2004) *The Skilled Helper – A Systematic Approach to Effective Helping*, 7th edn. Thomson Wadsworth, Belmont, CA.

Houston, G. (1995) *Supervision and Counselling*, 2nd edn. The Rochester Foundation, London.

Hunt, P. & Hilsdon, M. (1996) *Changing Eating and Exercise Behaviour*. Blackwell Science, Oxford.

Prochaska, J.O. & DiClemente, C.C. (1986) Towards a comprehensive model of change. In: *Treating Addictive Behaviours: Processes of Change* (eds W.R. Miller & N. Heather). Plenum, New York.

Rollnick, S. & Miller, W.R. (1995) What is motivational interviewing? *Behavioural and Cognitive Psychotherapy*. 23, 325–334.

Sanders, P. (2002) *First Steps in Counselling*, 3rd edn. PCCS Books, Manchester.

Shohet, R. & Wilmot, J. (1991) The key issue in the supervision of counsellors: the supervisory relationship. In: *Training and Supervision for Counselling in Action* (eds W. Dryden & B. Thorne). Sage Publications, London.

Waskett, C. (1993) *Guidebooks for Counsellors – Counselling People in Eating Distress*. British Association for Counselling, Rugby.

Williams, S. (1993) *An Incomplete Guide to Referral Issues for Counsellors*. PCCS Books, Manchester.

Part 2

The Skills

In Part 2, I show how the attitudes and awareness explored in Part 1 underpin the communication skills of attending and reflective responding. I focus on the skill of attending to verbal and non-verbal communication, which form the foundation of active listening discussed in Chapter 5. In Chapter 6, I explore different types of verbal response and the effect each has on the listener, and introduce the reader to the skill of reflective responding. By using the skills of active listening and reflective responding the dietitian is able to take in information, demonstrate empathy and build a helping relationship. These skills also provide the means to confront another in a non-threatening way, as shown in Chapter 7. This chapter introduces the reader to other helpful interventions and demonstrates how skilful questioning can be used effectively in a helping relationship.

In Part 2, I show how a dietitian can train herself effectively by:

- observing non-verbal communication and noticing discrepancies and incongruities;
- being aware of the many factors which can interfere with listening;
- becoming more comfortable with silence and emotional distress;
- increasing her understanding of the profound effect that words and the way they are used can have upon another;
- using reflective listening skills to demonstrate to a patient that they have been heard and understood, and to help a patient clarify what they have said;
- reducing the doubts and anxieties associated with confrontation by skilful use of reflective responding and questioning and in so doing help someone change.

Chapter 5

Active Listening

'It is the province of knowledge to speak and the privilege of wisdom to listen.'

Oliver Wendell Holmes

In this chapter I discuss:

- The process of listening
- Attending – a way of demonstrating acceptance
- Barriers to attending
- Attending to non-verbal communication
- Discrepancies and incongruities
- Developing powers of observation
- Managing silences
- Mirroring
- Touching

The process of listening

It is often said that communication is a two way process – of speaking and of listening. Although knowing what to say and expressing this clearly is obviously important when giving dietary information, being able to listen to the patient is fundamental to the development of a helping relationship.

Listening is often thought of as a *passive* process – an opportunity to sit back and relax while the other person does the work of communicating what they want to say. As a passive listener we may find ourselves thinking of other things and switching in and out of hearing what is being said. We may feel bored or guilty that we are not taking in what the speaker is saying and vow to ourselves that next time we will concentrate harder. We may feel irritated that the other person is not saying more clearly what they mean, that they are being long-winded and uninteresting. For their part the speaker who does not experience being listened to feels undervalued and negated.

Active listening on the other hand is a dynamic process which involves the skill of *attending*, i.e. giving someone our wholehearted attention. When attending, the listener finds it easier to concentrate and comprehend and is less likely to experience boredom. The ability to attend or 'be there' for someone is a basic counselling skill which offers in-depth support. As a result the other person feels affirmed in who they are, and becomes more open and more able to listen attentively in return. In this way, greater understanding develops and the relationship becomes more co-operative. This chapter focuses on attending and examines how the dietitian can develop her skills of attending. Chapter 6 focuses on ways of responding which demonstrate that she has listened.

Attending – a way of demonstrating acceptance

When attending, the listener is demonstrating the core condition of acceptance, as described in Chapter 3. The extent to which she can do this for a particular person depends upon her ability to accept that the other person has a right to express their point of view and that this may or may not coincide with her own.

A listener who conveys acceptance is someone who is safe to talk to

Conveying acceptance is related to our ability to accept ourselves. The more accepting we are of ourselves the more able we are to be open

---

Exercise 5.1

Think of a time when you felt safe to talk to someone. Recall what the listener did. Make a note of what you remember.

Exercise 5.2

You may like to practise by talking to someone you feel safe with using the topics here. Note those that you feel uncomfortable talking about.

- Something I feel strongly about
- Why I chose my profession
- My strengths and qualities
- My hopes for the future
- My fears for the future
- My thoughts on death

with ourselves and others (Chapter 3). When we are more accepting of ourselves we become less concerned with what others may think of us and more able to pay attention to what they say.

Counsellors in training focus on becoming more open and comfortable with themselves so that they are more able to understand and accept those they are helping. Some aspects of this process of personal development are explored in Part 4.

Attending is giving someone our attention as fully as we can

When attending we focus on the other person by observing their verbal and non-verbal communication and forming an impression of their attitudes and feelings. Attending also involves being aware of our own non-verbal communication which reflects our thoughts, feelings and attitudes. The more prejudiced we are, the more fearful or angry about something or someone, the more this will leak out in our non-verbal communication despite efforts to mask it. The more genuinely relaxed and at ease we are the more able we are to respond helpfully.

The following acronym (adapted from Egan (2004)) acts as a checklist to guide the dietitian in non-verbal communication when attending to another:

S   facing the other person as *squarely* as is comfortable
O   adopting an *open* posture
L   *leaning* a little towards the other person
E   maintaining *eye contact* without staring
R   keeping as *relaxed* as possible.

Barriers to attending

Many factors can interfere with our attempts to attend fully. Exercise 5.3 is designed to increase awareness of some of these. Lack of eye contact is one way in which we indicate that we are not listening and this has a profound effect on the person who is talking. When patients do not have eye contact with the dietitian they are likely to stop after a short while or may persist using a variety of means to attract the dietitian's attention. A barrier develops between patient and dietitian as the patient realises that they are not being listened to. This may occur when the dietitian is unable to maintain eye contact while simultaneously listening and writing down details of the diet history.

Exercise 5.3

With a colleague or friend, take it in turns to talk about an incident in your day, for example your journey to work. As a listener indicate in as many ways as possible that you are *not* listening. Take about three minutes each. (You may find it difficult to keep it up for this long.) Share with each other what you did, how you felt and what you were thinking, both when you were the listener and the speaker.

Now take it in turns to talk about something else, for example your plans for tomorrow. As the listener be as attentive as you can. Allow three minutes each and afterwards share again your thoughts, feelings and actions, both as the speaker and the listener.

Other factors which create a barrier between listener and speaker can be categorised under three headings:

- environment
- events and emotions
- echoes within.

Environment

Environmental factors, such as time constraints, temperature, humidity, noise, the room we are in and the seating available can all play a part in facilitating or hindering giving another person our full attention.

Events and emotions

Events can set in motion a train of thoughts and give rise to a variety of emotions. For example, the dietitian may feel pity, compassion, sadness, irritation, possibly anger, probably fear, maybe even horror when a patient talks about their illness. An emotional response may also be triggered if the dietitian notices something unexpected, such as a facial disfigurement or a limb missing. As a result her attention becomes focused on her own thoughts and feelings and she is unable to attend fully to what the patient is saying. Patients may explain details of relationships and activities that are outside the dietitian's experience. The dietitian may have strong opinions on the rights and wrongs of these and her beliefs and prejudices can become a barrier to listening. The extent to which her emotional response becomes a barrier to listening depends upon the intensity of her emotion.

Events may happen to the dietitian resulting in her being unable to give a patient her full attention. For example, if the dietitian witnessed an accident on the way to work and has not been able to talk about it to anyone, her shock and upset is likely to occupy her attention and limit her ability to give her attention to her patient. Similarly, an unresolved problem or conflict with someone else can gnaw away at the back of the dietitian's mind and the resultant anxiety can prevent her being fully present for her patient.

Echoes within

Echoes within are the thoughts we may have when we are listening to someone else. Although we may or may not be aware of them, they precede and colour our verbal response and influence our non-verbal communication. These internal echoes are often in the form of criticism, either of ourselves or of the other person. The following are some examples of thoughts which may be familiar:

- 'Surely that's not true.'
- 'They don't stand a chance of losing weight.'
- 'They're wasting my time.'
- 'It's useless giving them this advice.'
- 'That's a stupid thing to say.'
- 'Of course the trouble with this patient is . . .'
- 'What advice can I give now – they've tried everything – it's hopeless.'

In becoming more aware of these echoes and what they mean to her, the dietitian can begin to recognise and understand the ways in which they influence her communication with others.

Exercise 5.4

Take a piece of paper and a pencil. Sit quietly with arms and legs uncrossed. Close your eyes. Be aware of your breathing. Now focus on the sounds around you. Be aware again of your breathing. Now focus your attention inwards. As you become aware of a thought write it down. Your thoughts may well be judgements (criticisms or agreements) about what you have just read.

Attending to non-verbal communication

The voice

We speak with various accents and dialects and at different speeds. Voices are capable of a wide range, volume, pitch and tone. We express emotional states through our voice. When hearing someone's voice we make assumptions about them which may or may not be accurate (Exercise 5.5). For example, if someone is talking unnecessarily loudly, we may assume they are angry. However, on the one hand they may think the person they are talking to is hard of hearing. On the other hand they may be hard of hearing themselves and not realise the volume they are using. They may intend someone nearby to overhear or they may be in the habit of raising their voice and are unaware when this is unnecessary. If someone is speaking too quietly it is easy to assume they are shy and lacking in confidence. Whatever the reason, the speaker's voice affects the listener who may feel irritated, anxious or sympathetic.

Exercise 5.5

Focus your attention on someone's voice. How would you describe the volume, tone and pitch? Notice the speed of delivery, intonation, dialect and accent. What picture have you built up of this person?

Eye contact

Eye contact is used to send and receive information, show attention and interest. We use it to synchronise when to speak and when to listen. Eye contact also reveals attitudes. When we look into someone's eyes we may detect warmth or fear. In the former the pupils are dilated, in the latter the pupils contract. We spend 25–75% of the time looking at one another and look nearly twice as much while we are listening as talking. Eye contact can be unpleasant when strong emotions are aroused, if the topic is difficult or intimate or if there are other things to look at especially when these are relevant to the conversation such as a leaflet or diet sheet.

Exercise 5.6

Experiment with using more eye contact, then using less eye contact. Notice your reaction and that of the people you are talking to.

Facial expressions

The seven main facial expressions are happiness, surprise, fear, sadness, anger, disgust and interest. We are fairly aware of our facial expressions and can control them, although we may communicate the emotion through another part of our body. Smiling expresses happiness. It can also be used to ridicule, reassure or cover uncomfortable emotions. A genuine smile conveys warmth and openness.

Exercise 5.7

Be aware of facial expressions. Do you think they are genuine or assumed because they are what seems most appropriate to the situation?

Appearance

Appearance can convey social status, attractiveness and occupation. It expresses something about our attitude to ourselves and our environment. Many facets of appearance vary with changing fashions. Clothes, hair, skin and physique all communicate something about us. We 'carry' clothes differently depending on our attitude or the way we feel. They can show rebelliousness or conformity.

Posture

Posture indicates how tense or relaxed we are. Standing or sitting in a relaxed and upright position when listening indicates confidence. This in turn instils confidence in the speaker that they are being listened to. When listening we show interest by leaning slightly towards someone. By adopting a more open and relaxed posture we invite interaction and encourage others to be more open and accepting.

Exercise 5.8

Notice how posture changes in different situations and with different people.

Gestures

Gestures and body movements have been defined by Desmond Morris (2002) as any action which sends a visual signal to an onlooker. Gestures add meaning by displaying, pointing and illustrating. We use them to show agreement or disagreement, to describe, explain or question something, and to represent ideas and express feelings.

> **Exercise 5.9**
>
> When next listening to someone, notice what gestures they use and what these indicate to you.

Discrepancies and incongruities

It is important to place observations in context. A single gesture, for example clenching a fist, may not be of much significance on its own, but together with a reddening of the face, a pursing of the lips, a tightening of the facial muscles and a tensing of the shoulders, indicates someone who is experiencing a strong emotion. When words reinforce this non-verbal communication, for example, 'I wanted to throw the plate at him', we are left in little doubt that the patient felt angry. However, if the non-verbal communication indicates one emotion (e.g. the patient smiles) and the verbal communication another (e.g. anger as when saying 'I wanted to throw the plate at him'), the listener is likely to feel confused. We are more likely to believe the non-verbal message than the verbal. In the above example the skilled listener would probably conclude that the speaker was angry yet was not acknowledging this.

Incongruities also occur between a communication and the context in which it occurs. For example, a patient who has just received bad news may say 'I'm OK' with a fixed smile on their face when asked how they are feeling, leaving the dietitian unsure how to respond. Observing discrepancies and incongruities is fundamental when using counselling skills.

Developing powers of observation

We inform one another about our attitudes and emotions and present ourselves to the world through our non-verbal communication, which may support or conflict with any verbal communication. When there is a discrepancy we tend to believe the non-verbal rather than the words which are said. Attending therefore means listening with eyes as well as ears. Observations are made from what we see or hear, as for example 'I notice you are smiling' or 'I hear you say you are pleased that you have lost weight.' Helpful responding requires skilful use of observations (Chapter 6).

When using counselling skills it is important to distinguish between *observation* and *interpretation*. Observations are what we see or hear; interpretations are what we think and are based on assumptions and conclusions which may or may not be accurate. Interpretations form the basis of any judgements we make; for example, the dietitian may notice a patient is smiling (observation), think that this person is not taking her advice seriously (assumption), decide that the patient does not care about the diet (conclusion) and say, 'You haven't lost much weight have you?' (judgement implying the patient should have done better). Noticing when she moves from observation into interpretation is useful to the dietitian when deciding how to respond (Chapter 6).

Managing silences

People stop talking when they are unsure how to proceed, when they are struck by a thought that they have not yet articulated, or when they are experiencing a feeling which they are unsure of expressing. They may be assessing how safe they feel to express themselves. As the listener, the dietitian may feel uncomfortable if a silence lasts more than a few seconds and may either withdraw into herself or feel compelled to say something. As she searches for something to say she is likely to feel more anxious. She may think she should say something, that it is her responsibility to take charge of the situation. She may feel things are slipping out of control or think that she should keep the conversation going. She may want to protect the speaker from discomfort. One way in which she may cope with her anxiety is to come in quickly with a series of questions, so breaking the silence.

When the dietitian responds prematurely she crowds the patient and intrudes into their psychological space. This may produce temporary

---

Exercise 5.10

With a friend or colleague, practise sitting with each other in silence maintaining eye contact as you observe the non-verbal communication. Notice how long you can do this and feel comfortable. You could use an alarm to time this or invite a third person to do the exercise with you, taking it in turns to keep time for the other two. Be aware of what you are feeling and thinking as you do this. Share your experience of this exercise with each other. If you found it difficult and felt uncomfortable tell your colleague this.

You may want to do this exercise on your own. Have a paper and pencil at hand. Sit or stand in front of a mirror. Maintain eye contact with yourself. What do you notice? What are you feeling? What thoughts are you aware of? A useful way to debrief is to write down your experience of the exercise afterwards.

relief from discomfort for the dietitian, but the patient may feel upset at not being given enough time. Either way it is a missed opportunity for the dietitian to listen fully. Attending involves listening to the silences, being aware of our feelings as well as observing the other person. In attending, the dietitian may form a hunch as to how a patient may be feeling.

Being at ease with silence comes with practice. The more at ease she feels with silence the safer the dietitian will be perceived as a listener. When she allows the silence to take its course she gives the patient the choice of whether to speak.

Mirroring

Mirroring the other person's non-verbal communication develops the listener's understanding, demonstrates empathy and creates rapport. Mirroring is not the same as mimicking. Mirroring is based on a respectful desire to understand the other person, whereas mimicking is making fun of another.

We can mirror posture, gestures, facial expressions, and voice volume, tone and pitch. Mirroring is something we do naturally when we are getting on well with someone. We experience a warm feeling of rapport and feel understood. The times when we suddenly became aware that we are walking in step with someone or standing in the same position are spontaneous examples of mirroring.

Practitioners of neuro-linguistic programming develop the skill of mirroring to a fine art whereby they mirror breathing, eye movements and many finer points of non-verbal communication. Mirroring takes practice and at first may seem crude and obvious.

By mirroring someone's breathing we can get an idea of how they are feeling. When someone is anxious or fearful their breathing becomes more shallow, quite rapid and high in their chest. The more relaxed someone is, the slower and deeper the breathing.

Exercise 5.11

Practise mirroring as you listen to a patient talking. Notice their posture and discreetly adopt a similar one. As you focus on their gestures begin to mirror these by doing the same simultaneously. Keep your eyes on their face as you do so and maintain eye contact when you can. As they are speaking, their eyes will move in many directions. Your eyes need to be available to them when they seek you.

Touching

Touching is a powerful way of responding non-verbally to indicate caring, encourage trust and promote liking. We touch someone to guide them or attract their attention; for example, when we take someone by the arm to help them up or down stairs. There are strict social rules about touching. Infringing some rules clearly amounts to abuse. Other rules are unwritten and may be culturally specific.

There are codes of etiquette which if not adhered to can be interpreted as ignorance. The handshake is an example. The way in which we shake hands can tell us a great deal. If firm it inspires confidence; if limp and moist it indicates doubt and nervousness. Most people appreciate physical contact and find it reassuring. A hand on the shoulder, taking someone's hand in yours or putting your arm around someone's shoulder can say more clearly than any words that you are there for support in their distress. Some may find any form of touch threatening. It is important therefore to be aware of individual reactions to physical contact and to check before taking action if you are unsure how touch will be received.

Exercise 5.12

As a dietitian think of times when you have used touch to communicate with a patient. What was your purpose in doing this? What was the effect? Have there been occasions when you have felt moved to make contact through touch but have not done so? If so what held you back? If you had done so what do you think might have happened?

In this chapter, the importance of attending has been emphasised. The following chapter focuses on responding verbally and how this may help or hinder the development of a helping relationship.

References

Egan, G. (2004) *The Skilled Helper – A Systematic Approach to Effective Helping*, 7th edn. Thomson Wadsworth, Belmont, CA.

Morris, D. (2002) *Peoplewatching – A Guide to Body Language*. Vintage, London.

Chapter 6

Responding

'It takes two to speak the truth – one to speak and another to hear.'

Henry D. Thoreau

In this chapter I discuss:

- The effects of responding
- Types of response
- The purpose behind a response
- The power of language
- Reflective responding
- Mirroring language
- When and when not to reflect
- Self-disclosure

The effects of responding

There are times when we respond without fully understanding what has been said, hoping that our reply is appropriate. For example, patients may say 'yes' and nod in agreement as though they have understood when in fact they have not. The dietitian may not realise that the patient's subsequent lack of compliance is due to lack of comprehension. Instead, she may decide the patient is not motivated and so her responses will reflect her desire to motivate. Her attempts to do this will then be at cross-purposes with the patient's need for a clearer explanation. Thus, the way in which the dietitian responds affects her relationship with her patient and the outcome of an interview.

The effect of a response may be to arouse feelings of inadequacy and inferiority. When someone feels diminished they become defensive. As a result they may become over anxious to please or increasingly resentful and unco-operative. Patients are more likely to co-operate with the dietitian when she responds in ways which demonstrate her support. They are less likely to do so when she responds in ways which reinforce their sense of inadequacy.

Helpful responses facilitate the development of a therapeutic relationship and are concerned with empowering the other person. This chapter examines the different types of response and their effects on the dietitian's relationship with her patients.

Types of response

Some responses carry a higher risk than others of diminishing the other person. High-risk responses may hinder further communication and damage a relationship; low-risk responses are less likely to have this effect. Each type of response in Table 6.1 carries some risk. In addition to the words spoken there is the non-verbal communication associated with the response (see Exercise 6.1).

Table 6.1 Examples of different types of response.

Type of response	Example
Encouraging	'Right', 'mmm' 'uhuh'
Asking questions	'What do you eat normally?'
Making statements	'Eating too much is unhealthy'
Giving instructions	'Have three meals a day'
Making suggestions	'You could try . . .'
Giving advice	'If I were you . . .'
Challenging	'That's not right'
Confronting	'What do you mean?'
Criticising	'You're too fat'
Disagreeing	'No, you shouldn't . . .'
Giving solutions	'The answer is to eat less'
Praising	'Good for you'
Moralising	'You really should lose weight'
Threatening	'If you don't lose weight you'll need an operation'
Informing	'Poor diet is linked to heart disease'
Diverting from subject	'Do you like your job?'
Diverting onto own concerns	'I've been off sick myself'
Faking attention	'mm . . . I see . . . mm'

Exercise 6.1

Say each response in Table 6.1 in various ways by altering your tone and volume of voice. Imagine yourself as the receiver. How would you feel if someone responded to you in this way? Categorise the responses into high, medium, low risk of creating a barrier between speaker and receiver.

Low-risk responses

Encouragers are ways in which the listener can indicate interest and willingness to listen. As a result the speaker feels encouraged to talk further. Some examples are:

- The head nod.
- 'Um-hmm . . .'
- 'Yes.'
- 'Tell me more.'
- 'And . . .'
- 'Really?'
- 'And then . . .'

Overuse of encouragers can be a hindrance and an irritation to the speaker. We may not be aware of the frequency with which we use this form of response. It can become a habit or an unconscious way of expressing our impatience.

Opening statements invite the other person to talk. Some examples are:

- 'Would you like to talk more about it?'
- 'I'd like to hear what you have to say.'
- 'There seems to be something bothering you.'

Moderate-risk responses

- Asking questions
- Making statements
- Non-specific praising.

Much depends on the frequency with which questions are asked and the manner in which they are delivered, as well as the purpose behind them (Chapter 7). All questions are confrontational to some extent and so carry some risk of creating a barrier. Comments or statements are ways of expressing personal opinion, for example, 'I think that . . .' or 'In my opinion . . .' or 'I've read that . . .'. When not prefaced by 'I' the response carries a greater risk of being perceived as opinionated or patronising.

Although praise is designed to be encouraging, it can be perceived as patronising when it is non-specific. For example 'Good', 'Well done', 'Haven't you done well' offer non-specific praise. The risk of being perceived as patronising can be minimised by expressing praise specifically, for example, 'You are eating a healthier diet now you are eating more fresh fruit and vegetables'.

High-risk responses

High-risk responses are commonly used by those wanting to help others. The responses are authoritative in nature rather than facilitative and establish a relationship which encourages the patient to look up to the dietitian for evaluation rather than the dietitian supporting the patient to discover their own solution. High-risk responses include:

- Reassuring
- Giving instructions
- Giving advice
- Giving solutions
- Making suggestions
- Informing
- Persuading.

When the patient asks for information, suggestions, instructions or advice, responses in this category are effective. However, when such responses are unrequested the patient may perceive the dietitian as superior, may feel resentful and unwilling to co-operate, and may have thoughts such as 'Who does she (the dietitian) think she is'. Dietitians need to give information. However, an assumption may be made that the patient knows nothing about the subject. The dietitian then proceeds to give what she considers necessary information. This often results in her giving long explanations in her efforts to cover all the points. This increases the risk of the patient not listening, as much of the explanation seems irrelevant. The dietitian who makes a point of finding out first what information the patient wants can save herself and the patient a lot of time.

We often use persuasion when other methods, such as making a suggestion or giving an instruction, have failed to get us the outcome we want. If asked to explain why we are doing this we often say 'It's for their own good'. However, this means of communication has a high risk of creating a barrier between those concerned. The person who receives the communication may seem acquiescent at first but more than likely will feel confused and annoyed, if not immediately, then later. Many examples of this sort of interaction occur between parents and children, for example when a mother anxious to get a child to finish a meal, says 'You want to watch TV and your programme starts in five minutes so you'd better get a move on'. The child begins to eat then slows down. The mother then says 'Come on now – just finish it then you can watch TV'. In an interview with a patient a similar interaction occurs as follows:

DIETITIAN: (*anxious to motivate the patient*) If you want to lose weight before the wedding we need to start you on your diet straightaway.
PATIENT: Yes it's only six months away now. I'll try really hard this time. The only problem is I'm going on holiday next week so I won't be able to start until I get back.

As in the earlier example of the mother and child, the dietitian is then likely to resort to further manipulation which may take the form of a threat.

DIETITIAN: You have lost a little weight which is really good but if you aren't strict with yourself from now on you won't reach your target before the wedding.

Some use persuasion as a way of trying to motivate someone. However, rather than motivated and encouraged, the other person is more likely to feel controlled and resentful. Persuasion is a manipulative tactic frequently expressed in the form of a threat, for example 'If you don't . . . then. . .'. Although patients may very much desire the goal they have set themselves, the fear and annoyance engendered by the manipulative communication may outweigh their desire and their motivation will not be sustained.

Very-high-risk responses

- Challenging
- Criticising
- Moralising
- Confronting
- Disagreeing
- Threatening.

Reactions to these responses are likely to be defensive. Although at the time the recipient may agree with the response, they may later feel upset. Their hurt and anger is likely to leak out in disguised ways, for example they may not keep future appointments, they may turn up late, they may blame the treatment and they may criticise the dietitian to others.
   The following responses also carry a very high risk of creating a barrier in communication as they give a message which says 'I don't want to listen to you':

- Diverting to another subject
- Diverting to own concerns
- Faking attention.

Any response carries a risk of creating a barrier between people. When communication breaks down or becomes difficult it is valuable to reflect upon the type of responses made and work out other ways of responding which carry less risk.

The purpose behind a response

The purpose behind a response may be complex and varied. Table 6.2 gives some examples. We may not be aware of our underlying purpose or intention although this will be conveyed in the way we express ourselves (Exercise 6.2).

Table 6.2 Examples of different purposes behind a response.

Response	Purpose
'How do you do'	Establish friendship
'I'm the senior dietitian'	Establish status
'Yes . . . if that's all right with you'	Gain approval
'Sugar is a source of carbohydrate'	Give information
'Why did you do that?'	Curiosity
'I'm not sure I'm available then'	Be non-committal
'You can never rely on them to . . .'	Blame someone
'What will you gain from eating more healthily?'	Motivate someone

Exercise 6.2

Recall a recent interview with a patient. Remember as much as you can of how you responded. Reflect on your purpose in the interview.

Being more aware of her purpose helps the dietitian to become clearer in her communication and her responses are likely to be more open and direct. As a result the patient is less likely to feel confused and manipulated.

The power of language

The words we use can have as great an effect as the type of response. They can serve to form clear communication, or create misunderstanding and confusion. Effective use of language can help build a co-operative, rewarding relationship and ill-considered words can undermine and damage. Many people are aware of the misunderstandings which can result from the use of jargon and this topic is covered more fully in Chapter 8. This section examines the use of simple pronouns such as 'we' and 'you' and the ways in which words can indicate failure and negativity or can create change and self-confidence.

'We' and 'you' are frequently used to convey membership of a group or to speak on another's behalf. A dietitian could understandably feel confused when a patient, asked how frequently they eat a particular food, replies, 'We always have a large one once a week'. Who is 'we'? How many are included in 'we'? How is this divided? The more vague the reply, the more the dietitian will want to clarify what the patient has said. The use of 'we' and 'I' by the dietitian and the effect of this on the patient are examined in Chapter 8.

We develop patterns of speech which can convey an attitude of success or failure (Stewart & Joines 1987). Both dietitian and patient may talk about achieving a successful outcome using the language of failure, for example 'can't', 'shouldn't', 'have to', 'need', 'try'. A first step in changing such a speech pattern is to become more aware of the words used currently and their implications. For instance 'can't' implies 'being unable to', 'shouldn't/should/have to/must/ought' all imply a lack of choice and a handing over of power to another. Recognising and replacing these words with ones which convey ability, possibility and choice are an important part of developing a sense of resourcefulness and empowerment. The following example shows how a dietitian could do this:

> PATIENT: I *should* go on a diet. I *need* to lose weight.
> DIETITIAN: You *could* change your diet and be the weight you *want* to.

The way we use language can indicate lack of confidence. *Tag questions*, which are statements with questions added at the end, are an example. 'You know how much I want to lose weight, don't you?' is a tag question which indirectly invites the listener to agree or reassure (Morgan 1996). Dietitians may find it useful to reflect on their own use of tag questions and how these can communicate their lack of self confidence.

Instructions can be phrased in the negative by using 'don't' or in the positive by stating the desired behaviour. Although our intention in using 'don't' may be to reinforce the seriousness of the message, the use of the negative injunction focuses the attention of the listener, making it difficult to pay attention to anything else. When told 'Don't think of pink elephants' most people immediately conjure up an image of a pink elephant. People seem to respond more co-operatively when messages are phrased as a positive instruction (Morgan 1996). It is likely that patients who are told 'Learn how to make small changes in your diet' will heed the instruction more than those who are told 'Don't lose weight too quickly'.

Dietitians can therefore foster a climate which encourages change by paying close attention to the language used by both the patient and themselves. As the dietitian becomes more aware of the effect of language she is more likely to want to develop other ways of responding.

Reflective responding

Reflective responding is an effective way of demonstrating understanding and acceptance and of creating an environment in which change can take place. When the listener reflects back to the speaker what has been said, she is acknowledging that she has heard, accepted and understood. The speaker, on hearing the reflection, feels validated (Chapter 3). Reflecting leads to greater understanding because in the process any uncertainties are clarified. Reflecting is particularly useful when there is a problem, when something is unclear and needs clarifying and when someone is upset. Reassuring or suggesting what someone could do to feel better both carry a high risk of closing down on the relationship.

In the following example a dietitian uses a reflective response.

> PATIENT: I went out for a meal at the weekend and blew my diet. I have been trying ever so hard since but it's really difficult. It's the same when I go on holiday – I get so easily tempted. I don't know whether it's worth it.
> DIETITIAN: You find it very hard to keep to a diet and are wondering if it's worth the effort.
> PATIENT: Yes. I wonder if I'll ever lose weight.

If the reflection is inaccurate the speaker will respond in such a way as to clarify the misunderstanding as below.

> PATIENT: I went out for a meal at the weekend and blew my diet. I have been trying ever so hard since but it's really difficult. It's the same when I go on holiday – I get so easily tempted. I don't know whether it's worth it.
> DIETITIAN: You're wondering if it's worth going on holiday.
> PATIENT: No that's not what I meant. It's like . . . well . . . I doubt if I'll ever lose this weight. . . .

The technique of reflecting

When considering how to reflect there are a number of ways in which we can do this. One is to *repeat word for word* what has just been said. For example:

> PATIENT: I do try to keep to my diet.
> DIETITIAN: You are trying to keep to your diet.

Another way is to *repeat key words*, that is words that have seemed particularly significant.

PATIENT: I've tried absolutely everything. I don't know what to do next.
DIETITIAN: (*with emphasis*) Everything?
PATIENT: Maybe not everything. Perhaps there is something I could try?

Another way is to put into our own words what someone has said, that is *to paraphrase* as shown in the example below.

PATIENT: I have breakfast every day and then I don't have anything else until the evening. By that time I'm really hungry so I have a big meal then.
DIETITIAN: You have breakfast and then eat a large meal in the evening because you're very hungry by then.

Summarising is a way to reflect what has been said when the speaker talks for some time.

PATIENT: I went out for a meal at the weekend and blew my diet. I have been trying ever so hard since but it's really difficult. It's the same when I go on holiday – I get so easily tempted. I don't know whether it's worth it. I do try to keep to the diet though. I've tried absolutely everything. I don't know what to do next. I have breakfast every day and then I don't have anything else until the evening. By that time I'm really hungry so I have a big meal then.
DIETITIAN: You've tried hard to keep to your diet but when you get hungry in the evening or go out for a meal or are on holiday you find it too difficult and eat more than you need.

When considering what to reflect back to the speaker, the listener can focus on one of the following:

- the content of what has been said;
- the meaning this has for the speaker;
- the feeling that is expressed;
- the process that is taking place between speaker and listener.

When *reflecting content* the listener focuses on the words that have been said:

PATIENT: I do try to keep to my diet.
DIETITIAN: You are trying to keep to your diet.

When *reflecting meaning* the listener is assessing what she thinks this means to the speaker:

PATIENT: I do try to keep to my diet.
DIETITIAN: It would mean a lot to you to lose weight.

When *reflecting the feeling* the speaker has expressed, the listener takes into account non-verbal clues such as tone of voice and facial expression as well as the language the person has used:

PATIENT: (*frowning and speaking impatiently*) I do try to keep to my diet.
DIETITIAN: You feel frustrated keeping to a diet.

Reflecting process can be a greater confrontation to the speaker and is best used in an established relationship:

PATIENT: I do try to keep to my diet.
DIETITIAN: You are keeping to your diet some of the time but there are times when you don't?

The skill lies in developing a sense of the most appropriate choice to make when responding. Exercise 6.3 is an opportunity to practise reflective responses.

Exercise 6.3

Read each remark below and write your reflective response on a piece of paper. Consider more than one response, i.e. repeating word for word, selecting key words, paraphrasing. You may find it helpful to do this exercise with a colleague so that you can discuss your responses.

Example
PATIENT: You can't say no when people offer it to you, can you?

Responses:
(1)   You can't say no when people offer you something (reflecting word for word).
(2)   Can't? (reflecting key word).
(3)   You find it difficult to refuse when someone offers you something (paraphrasing).

Remarks:
'I've not been feeling too good since I last saw you.'
'My husband says I don't eat enough to keep a fly alive.'
'Everything I try giving him, he just won't eat.'
'It's not easy when all the family want something different.'
'I eat before I go out so I won't be tempted when I get there.'
'I have never had breakfast so I can't see me starting now.'

Repeat the exercise focusing on reflecting content, meaning, feeling or process.

Example
PATIENT: You can't say no when people offer it to you, can you?

Responses:
(1)   'Saying no is something you find difficult (reflecting content)'
(2)   'You think you have to accept when someone offers you something?' (reflecting meaning).
(3)   'You feel helpless in this situation?' (reflecting feeling).
(4)   'You're asking me if I find this difficult too?' (reflecting process).

The skill of reflecting

The dietitian may feel awkward when she first practises reflecting. Like any other newly acquired skill reflecting requires awareness, perseverance and practice. Fluency in paraphrasing and mirroring the emotional tone and meaning of what has been said are important sub-skills which the listener needs to develop if she is to avoid seeming artificial when she responds reflectively (Nelson Jones 2006). So far the focus has been on how to reflect short statements. However, much of the time people talk in 'paragraphs'. For example:

> PATIENT: I've just seen the doctor, he told me to come and see you for a diet. He's ever so nice, not the one I usually see but he told me not to worry and to come back in three months. I'll need to have transport though – I have to leave home at the crack of dawn and they go all round the houses to get here. It's such a nuisance. Can't I go to my own doctor?

Here the patient has given the dietitian some information ('I've just seen the doctor, he told me to come and see you for a diet'); also expressed some feelings (implied in the words 'It's such a nuisance'); posed a problem ('I'll need to have transport though – I have to leave home at the crack of dawn and they go all round the houses'); and asked a question ('Can't I go to my own doctor?') all in one speech. The dietitian has to decide what to focus on in her response. Does she pick one item or attempt to cover all? Does she choose the most important? And in deciding this is she selecting the one that seems most important to the patient (the transport), or the one that is of most concern to her (the diet)?

Summarising is a useful way to focus someone on the matter in hand. When the dietitian becomes aware that the patient is drifting off the topic she can refocus attention by summarising as shown here.

> DIETITIAN: The doctor said to come back in three months, in the meantime to see me about your diet. You're also worried about transport for next time and want to know if you can see your own doctor instead.

This response has the effect of confronting the speaker but not in a blaming or critical way. The dietitian is acknowledging the patient's concern and demonstrates caring and understanding without taking on responsibility for solving the appointment problem which is not her concern.

Focus on feelings

Many people find it difficult to express how they feel. Some have difficulty in finding words to describe their emotions. Some feel embarrassed about acknowledging sensations they do not find acceptable. Yet thoughts, feelings and behaviour are inextricably linked. When someone talks about something that is troubling or distressing them, the listener is likely to reassure or suggest what could be done for the person to feel better. However, as described earlier in the chapter, these ways of responding carry a high risk of closing down on the relationship. Sensitively reflecting how someone feels on the other hand demonstrates empathy and at a greater level than reflecting the content of what someone has said. In order to be able to demonstrate this we need to be able to recognise and put a name to the feeling that is being expressed. Identifying feelings can be easier when we consider them under the four categories of anger, fear, sadness and joy (Exercise 6.4).

Exercise 6.4

Take a piece of paper and divide it into four columns. Head one 'Anger', another 'Fear', another 'Sadness' and the fourth 'Joy'. Then write down as many words, phrases and behaviours as you can think of in each column.

We have many, varied ways of expressing feelings, as shown below:

- In words, for example 'I feel good', 'I feel angry', 'I'm scared'.
- In phrases, for example 'I'm on top of the world', 'I've been really down in the dumps'.
- By describing behaviour, for example 'I want to jump for joy', 'I felt like slamming the door'.

When reflecting feelings we can reflect the word used by the speaker, for example:

- 'I was annoyed because I missed the bus.'
- 'You felt annoyed.'

Or we can reflect the feeling implied in the phrase or behaviour described by the speaker as shown in the two examples below:

- 'I was really put out because . . .' becomes 'You felt annoyed because . . .'
- 'It made me see red when . . .' becomes 'You felt angry when . . .'

It is important to recognise the degree of intensity that the speaker is feeling and to reflect at the same degree of intensity. If someone says they are extremely annoyed it is not very helpful to them to reflect that they seem a trifle vexed!

When recognising how someone is feeling we take into account non-verbal clues such as smiling (joy), clenched fists (anger), looking down (sadness). Culturally we are not encouraged to express feelings and so we learn to mask them. When observing non-verbal clues we form hunches about how someone is feeling. A tentative reflection is a way of checking if this hunch is accurate. The tentative nature of the reflection can be conveyed by intonation, as for example 'You seem angry about that?'. This is an advanced empathic response (Chapter 3) and requires experience to use effectively. When used clumsily the other person will react defensively.

Mirroring language

We can mirror language as well as non-verbal communication. In neuro-linguistic programming (NLP) researchers have recognised that people predominantly use words from one of three categories to represent the way in which they think (O'Connor & Seymour 2003). These categories are 'visual', 'auditory' and 'kinaesthetic'. A few examples are given in Table 6.3.

Table 6.3   Examples of words in each category of expression.

Visual (see)	Auditory (hear)	Kinaesthetic (feel)
Appear	Overhear	Affected
Demonstrate	Hear	Feel
View	Listen	Rush
Look	Report	Sensitive
Notice	Tell	Stress
Watch	Mention	Touch

When using words in the same category as the other person we are literally speaking their language. We speak directly to them, thus avoiding some of the problems which arise from differences in understanding. The following is an example of a patient using visual language and the dietitian reflecting in the same language:

PATIENT: I always *watch* what I'm eating but I haven't lost any weight to show for it.

DIETITIAN: You keep *an eye* on what you eat but haven't noticed a change in your weight.

The dietitian has responded using visual language. Speaking the same language is something we all do naturally when we are in rapport. Using it consciously is a way of creating rapport. Notice the difference in rapport building when the dietitian responds using a different language.

> PATIENT: I always *watch* what I'm eating but I haven't lost any weight to show for it.
> DIETITIAN: You eat what you *feel* you should but this hasn't affected your weight.

When and when not to reflect

There are times when reflective responding is helpful and times when it is not. Reflective responding is useful when:

- someone expresses a concern;
- there is a problem;
- something is unclear and needs clarifying;
- someone is upset;
- there is a difference of opinion;
- you are presented with something unexpected.

Reflecting is valuable to do before you argue or criticise (Bolton 1986). When this takes place, greater understanding is gained before expressing an opinion. Bolton also advocates reflecting before taking action, by paraphrasing or summarising what has been discussed until agreement is reached about what is to be done.

It is not helpful to use reflecting when we are tired, rushed, frustrated, stressed or anxious and when we have too much on our mind to give our attention fully to another. Reflecting is a way of responding which reflects our attitude to another as being a human being worthy of respect and acceptance, who has the potential to find their own solution. It is therefore not useful or effective to use reflecting skills with those for whom we are not able to provide these core conditions (Chapter 3).

Reflecting requires us to be open to accepting the other person and ourselves. One way of becoming more open is to respond reflectively to oneself (Chapter 13). When we are unable to be open to another we can use listening as a way of hiding. This happens when we listen passively, letting the other person take charge of the situation. At such times when we do not want to engage with another we are not able to use reflective responding.

Self-disclosure

Talking about herself when interviewing a patient is something for the dietitian to consider carefully. What is her motive in talking about herself? Is it to establish friendship, feel better about herself, get the patient to comply with her instructions, gain the patient's approval, or to reassure the patient that he or she is not the only one with such a difficulty? Is the self-disclosure honest, appropriate and relevant to the patient? Is it for the benefit of the patient or the dietitian? What is the likely outcome of her self-disclosure?

The effect of self-disclosure may be to divert attention from the patient to the dietitian, as in the example below:

PATIENT: I haven't got much appetite – I don't think I'll be able to eat it all.
DIETITIAN: Don't worry, eat as much as you can. When I was in hospital I hardly ate a thing after my op.
PATIENT: Oh, what were you in for?

The interviewing time is for the patient not for the dietitian! Instead of using self-disclosure the dietitian could reflect as shown below:

PATIENT: I haven't got much appetite – I don't think I'll be able to eat it all.
DIETITIAN: You feel worried that you'll be expected to eat more than you can manage just now.
PATIENT: Yes, and then I don't want to try any of it.

As a result the patient has an experience of being heard and her lack of appetite accepted by the dietitian, who herself has a greater understanding of how the patient feels.

As well as diverting attention to the dietitian self-disclosure may result in patients feeling manipulated instead of empowered to act for themselves. The dietitian who makes up examples of eating behaviour and shares these with the patient as if they were her own, uses covert means in the hope of receiving an honest response. The dietitian may be tempted to do this when taking a dietary history, in the hope that she can convey acceptability to the patient of eating a particular food; for example, remarks such as 'We all eat chocolate biscuits from time to time. I know I do – once a packet is open you can't stop at just one or two can you?' Although her intention in making this remark is 'for the patient's good', the hidden message she conveys is 'I want to catch you out'. The patient is unlikely to feel safe enough with the dietitian to talk to her openly and honestly as the patient will sense the dietitian's lack of genuineness. This may not be apparent to the patient at the time but, as with all manipulative behaviour, it will be realised later. As a result distrust has been created in the relationship.

This chapter has identified different types of response and highlighted reflective responding as a skill which the dietitian can develop and use effectively in building a helping relationship with her patients. The next chapter examines the use of reflecting in dealing with confrontation as well as other ways of making helpful interventions and shows how these can be used in conjunction with reflective responding.

References

Bolton, R. (1986) *People Skills*. Prentice Hall, Sydney.

Morgan, L.B. (1996) Wordpower: using language to foster change. *Counselling*. 7, 55–59.

Nelson Jones, R. (2006) *Human Relationship Skills – Coaching and Self Coaching*, 4th edn. Routledge, London.

O'Connor, J. & Seymour, J. (2003) *Introducing Neuro Linguistic Programming*. Harper Collins, London.

Stewart, I. & Joines, V. (1987) *TA Today – A New Introduction to Transactional Analysis*. Lifespace Publishing, Nottingham.

Chapter 7

Making Helpful Interventions

'The Lion looked at Alice wearily. "Are you animal – or vegetable – or mineral?" he said, yawning at every other word.'

Lewis Carroll: *Through the Looking-Glass*

In this chapter I discuss:

- Towards a helping conversation
- Examining attitudes
- Providing the core conditions when making an intervention
- Asking questions
- Effective confrontation
- The timing and level of confrontation
- What to confront
- When the dietitian does not believe the patient
- Helping someone towards clearer thinking

Towards a helping conversation

A helping conversation consists of the helper not only demonstrating active listening and reflective responding as described in the previous two chapters, but also making skilful interventions. The nature, timing and content of these interventions are important if they are to perceived as helpful. As shown in the previous chapter, different types of response carry different degrees of risk of diminishing the other person and hindering the helping relationship. The manner in which a response is made also determines whether it hinders helpfulness or enhances the receiver's process. When skilfully applied, an appropriate intervention can help a person gain understanding, knowledge, insight and confidence. Such interventions can be classified as confronting, catalytic, supportive and informative (Heron 2001). A dietetic example of each type of intervention is given below:

- Confronting – 'If you could eat more healthily, what changes would you make?'.
- Catalytic – 'What would it mean to you if you were to lose weight?'.
- Supportive – 'You do matter, your health is important'.
- Informative – 'A persistent high blood level is a sign that something is not right'.

The purpose of catalytic interventions is to enable someone to think about something in a new way. In other words the intervention acts as a catalyst. The purpose of supportive and informative interventions, as their name implies, is to support and inform the other person. The person on the receiving end will also be brought face to face with the subject matter, that is they will be confronted with the topic or issue.

In many dictionaries confrontation is defined as meeting face to face although for many the word 'confrontation' is more associated with the idea of a head-on collision or conflict. There is often fear that a confrontation will be perceived as hostile and aggressive and so evoke a defensive and aggressive response. Such reactions occur when confrontations made clumsily and in anger, are perceived as uncomfortable and hurtful. Confrontation then, is generally perceived as something undesirable, even threatening rather than helpful and rewarding. This perception makes us wary of both giving and receiving such communications and so we may let opportunities pass by or make efforts to 'soften the blow', which can lead to misunderstanding and confusion. However, confronting a patient, that is helping them face something, is an essential part of enabling someone to change their behaviour.

Confrontation then is necessary and helpful and not harmful in itself although the way in which it is done can be. It is important therefore that interventions are made in a way that forms part of the helping process. When someone is brought face to face with something in a skilful and helpful way, the confrontation is likely to be experienced as constructive and helpful and to stimulate change. When an intervention is made with an attitude of enquiry and a desire to clear up a difficulty or to enable another person, it becomes less charged with anxiety. Effective confrontations are those which increase awareness, facilitate change and lead to completion of a task, growth in a relationship and personal development (Heron 2001). Clear, open and honest communication includes making interventions which are rewarding, stimulating, helpful, supportive and enlightening. They provide someone with an opportunity to learn something new. The ability of the dietitian to make effective confrontations is related to her *communication skills*, her *attitude* towards herself and others and the *manner* and *timing* of her intervention.

Examining attitudes

When examining her attitude towards confrontation it is important for the dietitian to consider her role. As a dietitian, on the one hand does she have permission to confront on the issue in question? If she exceeds her role she may be 'perceived as a bully, a do-gooder or a nag' (Heron 2001). If on the other hand she does not confront a patient, is she fulfilling her role to help that person change their eating habits? How much is her attitude towards confrontation affected by her fear of what might happen if she were to intervene? Dietitians who see themselves as facilitators may find effective confrontation comes more easily than those who see themselves as teachers or instructors. If a dietitian believes it is her role to facilitate and enable the patient to change their diet then she is likely to see any necessary confrontation as part of that process. In other words her confrontation is her 'best' way of responding to the patient in order to resolve or clarify a difficulty. If a dietitian sees her role as an adviser or teacher she is likely to feel a burden of responsibility to 'say the right thing', to give the 'right' instructions or advice. Her anxiety that she may get it wrong understandably makes her wary of confronting a patient.

Fear of what might happen

When feeling anxious about confronting someone, many people behave either manipulatively or aggressively. Initially they may try an indirect approach and do what they can to manoeuvre the other person in the direction they want. If this does not work they may pluck up courage to deal with the situation more directly. Phrases such as 'taking the bull by the horns' and 'tackling it head-on' come to mind. Stress levels increase and the belief that confrontation is difficult, anxiety provoking and unpleasant is reinforced.

Dietitians may fear that those they confront will perceive them as hostile and react by dissolving into tears or becoming verbally or even physically abusive. Although indirect and devious ways may prevent obvious distress, the patient who has been confronted will probably realise later that they have been manipulated. They may then feel irritated and confused and be doubtful about making a change. The following example, in which a dietitian is advising a patient on fluid restriction, illustrates this.

PATIENT: I try not to drink too much.
DIETITIAN: (*smiling and speaking brightly*) You mustn't drink a lot. It's important with your condition that you only have a litre of fluid a day. This may be difficult but once you get used to it you'll manage fine.

PATIENT: (*wondering how much a litre is*) . . . Mmm . . . I'm sure you're right. I'll have to get used to it.
DIETITIAN: (*wanting to be reassuring*) Oh there's no need to start unless the doctor tells you.
PATIENT: (*feels confused*) So I don't start now?

When confrontation is unclear, misunderstandings can accumulate until feelings reach such a level of intensity that someone feels compelled to say something or take some action. The subsequent effects on the relationship can be considerable.

Our point of view

It is difficult to make a helpful confrontation when we are unable to distance ourselves sufficiently to see any other point of view, although many people feel easier about confronting someone only when they are sure of their point of view and able to stand their ground in the event of an argument. Having a fixed point of view makes it difficult to listen to another person without risking loss of face. When one person is convinced their point of view is the only one worth consideration, confrontation easily becomes a conflict.

When two people share the same point of view they can reinforce each other in being 'right' and so make it more difficult for either to consider alternative possibilities and opportunities for change. We can confront one another most effectively when we are open to understanding and accepting another point of view at the same time as knowing our own.

Towards helpful confrontation

When an intervention is made in a spirit of wanting to clarify understanding, or to help another consider a different way of thinking, it becomes an invitation to change. The other person is less likely to feel obliged to defend themselves and therefore is more able to perceive the intervention as supportive. As a result they are more likely to be motivated to act. The following is an example of a dietitian confronting a patient in this way.

DIETITIAN: (*summarising what patient has said*) From what you tell me, cutting down on alcohol seems a big sacrifice at the moment as drinking is a way you deal with your stress.
PATIENT: What else can I do? If I didn't have a drink now and again it would all get on top of me.
DIETITIAN: (*paraphrasing*) You're not sure how else to cope. (*gives information*) There are other ways to manage stress. (*opens up an opportunity to*

give more information) If you would like to know more I can give you some information.

PATIENT: Yes. That might give me some new ideas.

Providing the core conditions when making an intervention

When our attitude to confrontation is based upon a desire to clarify understanding, showing respect for another and for ourselves, we are able to confront and simultaneously demonstrate our empathy, acceptance and genuineness. For example, when a patient complains to the dietitian about the hospital food yet the nursing staff have assured her that the patient eats the meals provided, the dietitian could demonstrate her genuineness by saying to the patient:

DIETITIAN: The nurses tell me you are eating well yet I am puzzled because you tell me that you dislike the food.

Here the dietitian has confronted the patient without attaching any blame either to the patient or the nurses, thus demonstrating her acceptance. She has expressed her genuine feeling of puzzlement at the apparent contradiction. On hearing this, the patient has no need to be defensive and has an opportunity to explain more fully if he wishes.

In the following example a patient explains that he finds it difficult to refuse the food served by his wife. The dietitian helps the patient face the problem through demonstrating her empathic understanding.

PATIENT: When I get a plateful in front of me, I just can't say no.
DIETITIAN: (*gently*) You can't?
PATIENT: Well . . . it's just so difficult . . . I don't want to hurt her feelings after she's gone to so much trouble.
DIETITIAN: (*reflecting*) You're worried she'll be upset if you don't eat it once she's cooked it for you?
PATIENT: I suppose the best thing would be to tell her before she starts cooking.

Gently reflecting the key word 'can't' in a questioning way brings the patient face to face with his statement and invites him to examine what he has said.

Asking questions

Questions are the most commonly used interventions and many dietitians are unaware of how many they ask and the way in which they ask them or of their effect upon the patient. When questions focus on the concerns, intent and perspective of the person asking the question they become a barrier to communication (Bolton 1986). Questions can be facilitative or authoritative in nature. They can be investigative, probing, inquisitorial and manipulative. They can also be expressions of curiosity. Questions have a useful purpose in *checking understanding* and *assessing knowledge*. The way in which a question is phrased, the purpose of asking it and the type of questions asked, all have an effect on the other person.

Questions can be open or closed. Open questions invite the other person to talk about the subject in some detail and begin with words such as 'what', 'where', 'when' and 'how'. Open questions phrased in this way are examples of facilitative questions. They show interest and concern and are useful in opening interactions; for example, 'How are you?' is an open question used in everyday conversation.

Dietitians often ask 'How can I help you?'. This example of an open question can be effective in the opening stages of an interview with a patient. Open questions are an effective way of *focusing attention* on a particular topic, as in 'What did you have for breakfast this morning?'. Open questions can induce motivation. For example the dietitian may ask 'What would you like to be able to do as a result of losing weight?'. This catalytic intervention invites the recipient to think about what losing weight means to them. If the patient perceives herself safe enough to answer honestly she may take the opportunity to clarify her thoughts. If these are realistic and she receives acceptance not criticism, she is more likely to be motivated to take the necessary action. Thus, by asking open questions the dietitian encourages greater participation and invites the patient to express their opinions, attitudes and feelings. Although open questions may yield seemingly irrelevant material and place more demand upon the dietitian to listen, the fuller reply which they evoke allows for a more accurate assessment than is obtained through the use of closed questions.

Questions beginning with 'why' are frequently used to obtain the reason behind something. While this may be asked out of curiosity there is considerable risk that the person being asked the question will feel interrogated. They are likely then to come up with an answer which they think will satisfy the questioner, rather than an honest explanation. The dietitian who asks, 'Why don't you eat boiled eggs instead of fried?' is likely to get an evasive and defensive reply such as, 'Oh it's not me that has them fried, it's the rest of the family that like them this way. I always boil mine.' The dietitian is then faced with the dilemma of whether to believe the patient or not.

Closed questions invite a monosyllabic response such as 'yes' or 'no' and are useful for getting specific information. By asking questions which elicit a minimal answer the questioner retains control of the interview. However, even if the person gives more than a monosyllabic answer, they are unlikely to disclose much, particularly about their feelings. The reply to a closed question may also be misleading. A patient may answer 'Yes' in response to the dietitian asking 'Do you understand?' because this is what is expected, and in doing so they may imply a greater understanding than they actually possess. Closed questions inviting only a limited reply may provoke frustration in articulate patients.

It is important the dietitian is aware of her purpose in asking the question. Knowing this can help her decide whether to frame it as an open or closed question. A closed question is adequate if the dietitian knows specifically what information she requires. If she wants to encourage her patient to talk and think for themselves, and wants to ascertain general information, an open question is more likely to fit her purpose. The examples of confronting and catalytic questions on p. 87 illustrate this.

As she becomes more aware of the way in which she asks questions, the dietitian may be at a loss as to other ways to respond. When people give up their over-reliance on questioning they usually feel uncomfortable with the silences (Bolton 1986). The skills of active listening and reflective responding (Chapters 5 and 6) and assertive communication (introduced below), are valuable alternatives.

Effective confrontation

Effective confrontation involves:

- listening to the other person's point of view;
- stating the facts;
- being specific;
- speaking for oneself using 'I';
- skilful questioning.

The skills of active listening and reflective responding described in Chapters 5 and 6 clarify understanding and demonstrate listening to the other point of view. Stating the facts involves sharing observations and referring to actual events that took place. Phrases such as 'When you . . .' or 'When I . . .' (followed by the behaviour) or 'When (the event) happened I (noticed/thought/felt) . . .' are useful as a way to raise the subject. The skill in being specific is to keep to the behaviour in question. It can be tempting to generalise and add other situations and refer to other examples. This can lead to side-tracking and loss of impact. Speaking for oneself involves the skills of assertive communication (Chapter 13) and using 'I' as the pronoun not 'you'.

In the following example the dietitian who has thought about confronting the patient for some time has now decided to do so using the skills described above.

> PATIENT: (*having gained weight*) I always do that – lose some and then put it back on. It doesn't seem to make much difference coming here.
> DIETITIAN: (*reflecting*) You think there's not much point in coming here any more. (*stating her point of view*) As I see it we have been meeting for over a year now. During this time you have made some changes to your diet and lost weight although you have put some on in the past three months, overall you have lost weight. (*Invites patient to assess progress*) I am wondering what you have got from our meetings that has been helpful to you?

The timing and level of confrontation

Knowing that confrontation is likely to arouse anxiety in both herself and her patient, the dietitian will want to consider an *appropriate time* to make an intervention. When considering this she will be taking into account the quality of the relationship she has established with her patient and assessing her patient's ability to act upon her confrontation. In the following example a dietitian has been listening attentively and consciously using reflective responding for much of the interview. She is aware her patient uses phrases such as 'I can't . . .' and 'I'll never be able to . . .' followed by 'It doesn't really matter' and 'I'm fine really, I've always been like this'. The dietitian recognises these phrases as examples of discounting (Stewart & Joines 1987). We can discount:

- our ability to change, e.g. 'I can't (keep to a diet)';
- the possibility of change, e.g. 'It will never happen. (I'll never lose weight)';
- the significance of the event, e.g. 'It doesn't really matter (being clinically obese)';
- the existence of the problem, e.g. 'I'm fine. I've always had this (been overweight)'.

A confrontation may be ignored or deflected onto something else if someone is not ready to listen, with the result that no change takes place. As a general guideline it is effective to confront someone at the time or as near to this time as possible. The more time that elapses the more room there is for misunderstandings and anxiety to develop and details become less clear. If considerable time has passed, the other person may not even remember the occasion or issue in question.

The level of confrontation is important. If the confrontation is superficial it will be treated as insignificant. If the confrontation is too deep the person concerned will defend themselves in some way, for example by brushing it aside or denying their part in the situation, as in the following example.

> PATIENT: It's so difficult to refuse. I just can't say no to chocolate cake. I'm hopeless.
> DIETITIAN: (*briskly*) Have you thought of some assertiveness training.
> PATIENT: Oh no . . . I couldn't possibly.

The ability to assess the timing and level of an appropriate confrontation is closely linked with being empathic. The dietitian who focuses on providing the core conditions of empathy, acceptance and genuineness as described earlier in this chapter, will find that she is able to respond to her patient appropriately by using reflective responding or purposeful questioning.

What to confront

How does the dietitian know what to bring face to face with another? She can choose to confront how someone *feels*, for example their anxiety; how someone *thinks*, for example the accuracy of their knowledge; or how someone *behaves*, for example the fact that they missed their last appointment. Some more examples of different feelings, thinking and behaviour are given in Table 7.1.

It is important to confront one thing at a time. It is not helpful to confront someone with, for example, their incorrect knowledge about foods rich in saturated fat, the appointment they missed last week and their air of depression, all in one sentence! Given that there is so much to choose from how does the dietitian decide what to focus on? Her choice depends upon her awareness. As she listens to the patient she may become aware of their hesitant tone of voice, for example, and choose to focus on this by saying, 'You sound unsure when you say that'. She may notice a frown on the patient's face and wonder if they have understood. She could confront this by saying, for example, 'I'm not sure if I've explained myself clearly. Would you like me to go through it again?'

Confronting paradoxes, discrepancies and inconsistencies

The dietitian may be aware of a particular *paradox*, *discrepancy* or *inconsistency* in what the other person is saying; for example, she may

Table 7.1   Examples of different feelings, thinking and behaviour.

Feelings	Anger
	Concern
	Uncertainty
	Fear
	Frustration
	Sadness
	Disappointment
	Irritation
	Relief
Thinking	Knowledge
	Point of view
	Attitudes
	Expectations
	Beliefs
Behaviour	Missing appointments
	Expressing opinions
	Refusing to comply
	Crying
	Not talking
	Diverting onto another subject
	Not achieving a target
	Complaining about someone else
	Shouting
	Any non-verbal communication

realise the patient has contradicted himself. When the dietitian recognises a discrepancy she may feel confused and decide that the patient is lying or that she has misheard. She may ignore it and miss the opportunity to clarify what the patient said, or ask a series of questions in an attempt to establish the truth. Too many questions are likely to produce a defensive response. The dietitian can bring her observation to the patient's attention by using the phrase, 'On the one hand I hear you say . . . yet on the other you tell me . . .'. By highlighting the contradiction in this way she is confronting the patient in a non-threatening manner.

Another way to confront involves reflecting the inconsistency, as in the following example. The question mark indicates the dietitian's puzzlement rather than criticism.

DIETITIAN: (*with curiosity*) 'You say you had some last week yet earlier I thought you said you this was something you never ate?'

The dietitian has an opportunity to confront when a patient uses words such as 'never', 'always', 'everyone', 'no-one'. These are examples of words which define something in absolute terms. Such words are all embracing and exclude alternatives. When someone says, for example, 'I never eat (a certain food)' they may be dismissing occasions when they have. 'I always eat breakfast' similarly discounts any occasion when this meal was not taken. Use of such words can alert the dietitian, for they may imply that a patient is not yet open to change. The dietitian has an opportunity to confront the patient with what they have said by reflecting the key word, for example 'never' (Chapter 6). In so doing she is inviting the patient to think about what they have said.

Confronting issues

The dietitian may come across a situation in which she is aware of certain issues, such as a patient's lack of trust in the hospital food. For example, a patient is not eating his hospital diet despite efforts by the dietitian to make sure the food he likes is available. When the dietitian learns that the patient's wife is supplying him with food she assumes he is not willing to comply with his diet. She later learns about his religious background and she suspects that he does not trust the hospital to provide food that suits his beliefs. She has now replaced her initial assumption that he is deliberately being difficult because he is unconcerned about his diet, with the hunch that he does not trust the hospital to provide meals which are acceptable. She decides to confront him with this by first stating the facts and then sharing her thoughts, and she invites the patient to explain his point of view:

> DIETITIAN: The nurses tell me that you are not eating your meals except those your wife brings you and I'm wondering if this is because you don't like the hospital food.

When the dietitian does not believe the patient

'I don't believe you but I can't say that' is a thought which may occur to a dietitian as she listens to a patient, and it provides her with an opportunity to confront her patient in a constructive way. The following example demonstrates this.

> PATIENT: (*at appointment following return from holiday*) I had a wonderful holiday, good weather, great company and marvellous food. I was very good though – I kept to my diet all the time.
> DIETITIAN: (*not sure whether to believe this or not, decides to accept it at face value*) You enjoyed your holiday and kept to your diet throughout.
> PATIENT: Yes, I surprised myself but there was so much variety I could choose lots that is OK on my diet. I didn't feel I was going without.

DIETITIAN: (*hunch that patient is being honest*) There was a lot of choice and you didn't find your diet restricted you. I'm glad for you because holidays can be difficult times to be on a diet.

PATIENT: I know. I wondered if you'd believe me. I'm pleased you do but I wouldn't have been surprised if you hadn't.

This interview could have turned out differently as shown below. In both examples the dietitian focuses on reflective responding as a non-threatening way to confront the patient.

PATIENT: (*at appointment following return from holiday*) I had a wonderful holiday, good weather, great company and marvellous food. I was very good though – I kept to my diet all the time.

DIETITIAN: (*not sure whether to believe this or not, decides to accept it at face value*) You enjoyed your holiday and kept to your diet throughout.

PATIENT: Well, almost. You won't be cross will you if I tell you there was one occasion . . . on the last evening I had a real blow out but that was the only time.

DIETITIAN: (*decides to ignore the invitation to admonish or commiserate with the patient*) The last evening you decided not to limit yourself.

PATIENT: Yes, I paid for it though . . . had indigestion all night.

Helping someone towards clearer thinking

When the dietitian becomes aware that the patient is using phrases such as 'I can't', 'it doesn't matter' or words such as 'never', 'always' or recognises other examples of discounting (p. 93), she has an opportunity to help the patient change their way of thinking. As a result, feelings change and different outcomes are possible. The strategies to enable this to take place are encompassed in cognitive-behavioural therapy (CBT, described in Chapter 1) and can be helpful to the dietitian, both in her own personal development (Chapter 14) and in her work with patients. The following CBT strategies are useful to help a patient gain a different perspective and are appropriate when both patient and dietitian are working in Stage 2 of the helping process described in Chapter 4.

Recognising thoughts and distinguishing these from feelings

To be able to change our thinking we first need to distinguish our thoughts from our feelings. This is not so straightforward as it seems as much of the time we express feelings as thoughts and vice versa. For example when asked how they feel someone may reply 'I **think** I could do with a holiday'. When asked what they are thinking someone may reply 'I **feel** exhausted'. The dietitian who becomes adept at distinguishing thoughts from feelings can help her patient think, feel and behave differently.

What's going through your mind when you think that?

This is a useful question to ask a patient who is ready to gain a new perspective. When she asks this question the dietitian is inviting the patient to describe the thoughts that are occurring to him in association with a particular feeling or behaviour. Patients may find this difficult to articulate at first. Some may be willing to keep a record of their thoughts, associated with a particular behaviour, between appointments (an example of how this can be done is given in Exercise 15.5, Chapter 15). This exercise could usefully be incorporated into a food diary. Keeping such a record can help someone become more familiar with the process of identifying their thoughts. In the following example the patient is talking about how difficult she finds it to refuse food.

> PATIENT: I just wish I could say no when I'm offered a second helping but I can't.
> DIETITIAN: I'm wondering what is going through your mind when you think that?
> PATIENT: Oh . . . I don't know . . . I'm hopeless . . . I just haven't any will power.

As she listens the dietitian is identifying the extreme negative thoughts of 'I can't' and 'I'm hopeless'. In saying this the patient is discounting her ability to change by focusing solely on negative beliefs. Identifying this and replacing these negative thoughts with more realistic ones enables the patient to gain a different, less one-sided perspective. The dietitian now helps the patient do this as follows:

> DIETITIAN: When I hear you say 'I can't and I'm hopeless', I'm wondering if these thoughts are really true? And I'm thinking what if you were to replace those thoughts with more realistic ones. For example 'What if I could? Then what?'.
> PATIENT: I suppose I would feel less hopeless.
> DIETITIAN: (*summarising*) So when you're offered another helping you could say no and this would mean you would feel less hopeless?
> PATIENT: I suppose so. . . . .
> DIETITIAN: And if you felt less hopeless how would this affect your will power?
> PATIENT: I suppose I would then have a little.
> DIETITIAN: (*invites patient to practise*) How about imagining you are about to comfort eat and saying to me now 'I could say no'?

Patient nods and repeats the phrase hesitantly back to the dietitian saying she feels silly.

> DIETITIAN: (*acknowledging how patient feels*) Yes, it seems strange at first to hear oneself saying something you're not used to. How about having another go and speaking more firmly this time?

The dietitian then invites the patient to repeat her new way of thinking several times. Patients differ in their willingness to engage in this exercise. Although those who decline to participate will not have heard themselves utter a new thought they will go away with a greater understanding of how they could change their thinking. Patients who do take part are likely to say how strange they feel saying these unfamiliar words. The dietitian can encourage them by affirming each attempt.

Some other typical examples of negative thinking are given in Table 7.2. These examples can be replaced by more positive and realistic thoughts such as shown in Table 7.3.

Table 7.2   Typical examples of negative thoughts.

Negative thought	Assumption
'Now I've blown my diet completely'	There is no way forward
'I'll never be slim again like I was before'	I can't change
'I know you're going to tell me off'	I'm in the wrong again
'I just know I've put on weight'	I can't succeed
'I feel guilty I can't keep to a healthy diet'	I'm a failure

Table 7.3   Some examples of replacements for negative thoughts.

Negative thought	Replacement
'Now I've blown my diet completely'	'I've eaten more than I intended but I can have less this evening'
'I'll never be slim again like I was before'	'It may be difficult to lose weight but not impossible'
'I know you're going to tell me off'	'I have done the best I could given the circumstances'
'I just know I've put on weight'	'I will only know this when I get on the scales'
'I just can't keep to a healthy diet'	'Over the past week I've not done too badly'

By replacing negative thoughts with helpful positive ones we are not only being more realistic but also showing more compassion. Instead of putting ourselves down in a harsh and critical way, we can learn to talk to ourselves in the same compassionate way we would to a friend with a similar problem. In other words we can learn to be our own best friend! The following example shows how such self-compassion can be developed.

The mother of a child with sensitivity to cow's milk finds out her child has been given milk to drink at nursery school. She holds herself personally responsible for an event that isn't entirely under her control. As a result she feels guilt, ashamed and inadequate as a mother. She thinks 'It's all my fault. If I were at home instead of at work this wouldn't have happened'. Realising how she is thinking she now says to herself, 'The reality is that this has happened and could have done so whether I was at home or at work. What I can do now is think how I can reduce the risk of it happening again'.

We not only blame ourselves but also blame others, or the circumstances, for a problem and in so doing overlook the part we may have played. The following example shows a patient complaining to a dietitian.

> PATIENT:　'It's all the doctor's fault. If I'd been told to lose weight sooner I wouldn't have to wait so long for the operation'.
>
> DIETITIAN:　(*first identifies the blaming thought then uses reflective responding to invite the patient to reconsider*) 'You're thinking it is all the doctor's fault that you are having to wait so long for your operation'.
>
> PATIENT:　'I realise it is not all the doctor's fault but he could have sent me to see you sooner'.
>
> DIETITIAN:　(*paraphrasing*) 'You would have found it helpful to have had advice about losing weight at an earlier stage?'
>
> PATIENT:　(*now thinking clearly*) 'Yes. If I had succeeded in losing weight last year I might not have had so long to wait for my operation'.

When we blame ourselves or others we tend to use words like 'should' 'need', 'ought', 'must' and 'got to'. Thinking something or someone **should** be the way we hope or expect indicates that we are thinking in a demanding and inflexible way. The following are typical examples: 'I really should try harder to stick to my diet' and 'They should know by now not to give me things I shouldn't eat'. 'Should' statements may be directed towards others or oneself, to particular individuals or groups or the world in general and lead to frustration and anger. Some people think 'should' and 'must' statements are motivating to the other person. However there is a high risk that these statements will chastise and demotivate leading to a refusal to co-operate.

Another way in which we attach blame and evoke negative thoughts is when we define ourselves using an action or event and assume that what we do is who we are. For example a patient buys or eats an unsuitable food then thinks 'I'm stupid' or 'I am a fool'. This way of thinking arouses anger, depression and low self-esteem. As well as labelling ourselves we label others in a similar way, such as when someone behaves in a way we don't like we think of them as 'bad'. For example when a dietitian thinks a patient is awkward and demanding and then considers him to be a bad patient.

We can learn to think in ways which do not distort the reality by applying the following three steps:

(1) Identifying the negative way we are thinking
(2) Challenging the assumption that the negative thought is true
(3) Replacing the negative thought with a more appropriate one. For example 'should' statements can be replaced with 'it would have been better if I had . . .' or 'I prefer to . . .' or 'I aim to . . .'.

Here are some ways to help someone challenge their negative thought:

- helping them to list the reasons why this might not be true;
- asking questions, e.g. 'How do you know this?' 'What if this weren't so?';
- inviting them to think in terms of partial success rather than complete failure;
- asking them to rate, e.g. hunger, on a scale (1–10) helps someone to evaluate an event or feeling and make an assessment;
- inviting them to ask others if their thoughts and attitudes are realistic;
- reminding them that doing something idiotic or foolish does not mean they become an idiot or a fool;
- encouraging them to talk to themselves in a gentler, less emotionally laden way;
- helping them consider the many factors that may have contributed to their negative thinking.

Not all patients will be willing to change the way they think. However doing so can lead to a greater sense of fulfilment and possibility of change. The dietitian who is familiar with identifying, challenging and replacing negative thoughts for herself can incorporate these steps into her way of helping patients as shown in the examples above.

This chapter has examined the skills of questioning and, together with the skills of active listening and reflective responding described in the previous two chapters, shows how these interventions can be effectively applied to help a patient in the process of change. Although all the examples in Part 2 are related to the dietetic interview, dietitians will find it helpful to apply the principles in their interactions with others, for example with students. Part 3 focuses on the patient interview and demonstrates how these skills can be used in a variety of settings.

References

Bolton, R. (1986) *People Skills*. Prentice Hall, Sydney.

Heron, J. (2001) *Helping the Client*, 5th edn. Sage Publications, London.

Stewart, I. & Joines, V. (1987) *TA Today – A New Introduction to Transactional Analysis*. Lifespace Publishing, Nottingham.

Part 3

The Patient Interview

In Part 3, I show how the skills described in Part 2 can be used in dietetic practice. Chapter 8 focuses on developing a framework for the dietetic interview, consisting of three sections (beginning, middle and ending) and certain tasks within each section. The beginning section plays a significant part in creating an environment in which dietitian and patient can work comfortably together. First impressions are quickly formed by both patient and dietitian and assumptions made which affect their communication with each other. Setting an agenda and clarifying the time available and the limits to confidentiality establish boundaries which enable the dietitian to use her counselling skills effectively. The middle section of the interview includes assessing motivation to change the diet, forming a working agreement or contract, taking a diet history and giving dietary advice. When these tasks are accomplished using a person-centred approach, a relationship of trust, respect and individual responsibility develops. The chapter concludes with the process of closing the dietetic interview and how the dietitian can use the interview framework to review her work in a structured way.

Some particular issues of working with different groups of people, for example those who are bereaved, children, those whose cultural background differs from that of the dietitian and those with physical and mental health problems are addressed in Chapters 9–12. These are included to help the reader recognise and understand how:

- bereavement is part of adapting to any change and how grieving a loss evokes an intense mixture of thoughts and feelings and results in people behaving in many different ways;
- an awareness of the dynamics between the family members increases the dietitian's understanding of the child and his or her environment;

- cultural differences and attitudes can create commonplace mis-understandings, threaten human relationships and result in the ineffective use of time and resources;
- patient and dietitian reflect their attitudes about physical and learning difficulties and mental health in the way they communicate with one another. Anxiety, depression and deep-seated difficulties concerning the use and abuse of food require skilled help from dietitians and others.

Chapter 13 describes three interviews in which I show how dietitians can integrate into dietetic practice:

- the issues raised in Part 1;
- the counselling skills described in Part 2;
- the framework described in Chapter 8.

Chapter 8

Developing a Framework

' "I could tell you my adventures beginning from the beginning" said Alice a little timidly.'

Lewis Carroll: *Alice in Wonderland*

In this chapter I discuss:

- A framework for the interview

Beginnings

- The interview setting
- Preparing to provide a helping relationship
- First impressions
- Opening the interview

Middles

- Setting the agenda
- Assessing motivation

- Making a contract
- Taking a diet history
- Giving dietary advice
- Monitoring the relationship

Endings

- Closing the interview
- After the interview

A framework for the interview

Working within a framework helps the dietitian to contain and manage both her patient's anxiety (described in Chapter 2) and her own (described in Chapter 4). Anxiety can give rise to common problems in an interview (Table 8.1).

A framework also helps the practitioner monitor, review and learn from the interview. The framework described in this chapter is based on accepted practice in counselling and psychotherapy and has been

Table 8.1   Some examples of problems that can arise if anxiety is present.

Anxiety about	Problem
Available time	Pace – going too fast or too slow
	Rambling – on the part of the patient and/or the dietitian
Getting it right	Probing – excessive probing being perceived as intrusive
	Embarrassment (shame) – of either patient or dietitian
Pleasing another	Flexibility – too much or a lack of this
Safety/security	Issues about confidentiality and talking openly

applied to a standard dietetic interview. The interview has been broken down into three stages: beginnings, middles and endings.

Beginnings

The interview setting

Environmental factors such as temperature, humidity, noise and seating can either facilitate or hinder the dietitian in giving her full attention to the patient. Rooms in out-patient departments which are too warm, windowless or airless may be familiar to many. Some rooms have little privacy; others are so cut off from the main area that dietitians feel isolated. Patients can spend time wandering aimlessly in search of where to go and this increases their anxiety. Although environmental factors may be outside the dietitian's control, small changes can often be made which result in a more effective environment (Exercise 8.1).

Exercise 8.1

Think of your workplace. What environmental factors do you consider a barrier to listening? What changes would you like to make? You may find it helpful to list these under the headings of 'barriers' and 'possible changes'.

Position of desk

It is well recognised that a desk between two people is an obstacle to communication. Nowadays computers may add to the impedimenta on desk tops. Objects placed between dietitian and patient cut off some of the information communicated by each person; for example, if a desk is between her and her patient the dietitian is unlikely to notice the patient's foot tapping rhythmically. If she were to notice this she might interpret it as a sign of agitation and an indication that the patient is having difficulty listening.

Seating

We tend to sit opposite one another on either side of a desk if we want to compete or negotiate; side-by-side to co-operate; and diagonally opposite to discuss. If seats are identical there is no problem in deciding which one to take. If they are different the dietitian needs to assign one for herself and one for the patient. Should she have the more comfortable chair because, as the dietitian, she will be sitting in it throughout the clinic, or should she offer this to the patient? What is the likely effect on the patient and the relationship between them when the dietitian commands the superior chair?

Proximity and orientation

The closer and more direct (face to face) two people are, the more open they become to one another. On the one hand this may indicate intimacy; on the other hand one or the other may feel threatened. We show interest by leaning towards each other, yet if we lean too close we invade the other's personal space. Our willingness to allow someone to enter our personal space varies according to our relationship with them, the job we do and the culture we come from. Doctors, dentists and nurses, for example, are allowed to enter a patient's personal space because of the role they fulfil, whereas dietitians may not have the same permission. Having considered these aspects of the physical framework the dietitian needs to consider how able she is to provide a helping relationship (Chapter 3) and how her attitude may be influenced by the first impression she is forming of her patient.

Preparing to provide a helping relationship

The dietitian can prepare herself before an interview by allowing enough time to adjust the physical environment and giving herself time to reflect upon the following.

Practical

- Have I read the patient's notes?
- Do I need to speak to another member of staff (e.g. doctor, nurse, receptionist) before I see this patient?
- Do I need to set up the computer?
- What resources (e.g. diet sheets, information leaflets) do I need on hand that might be useful?

Personal

- How able am I right now to listen to this patient?
- How able am I to provide the core conditions of empathy, acceptance and genuineness?
- What is my agenda for this appointment?
- Am I able to set clear boundaries about time, confidentiality and further appointments?

Checking these points is a useful habit. The reader is recommended to refer to Chapters 3 and 4, where these points are discussed and examples are given of setting boundaries about confidentiality and time. There will be times when, for many reasons, the dietitian is not able to offer the patient much apart from answering questions and giving brief information. There will be other times when the dietitian realises that she can give the patient the support they need through using her skills of active listening, as described in Chapter 5.

First impressions

The first impression we form of someone happens very quickly in any meeting. During the 'safe talk' period we absorb a lot of information, mainly from the other person's non-verbal communication. Tone of voice, posture and facial expression give clues about a person's emotional state; for example, someone introducing themselves in a gruff tone of voice and with a frown on their face is likely to be perceived as irritable and ill at ease. Someone who is speaking in a warm tone and with a smile on their face is thought to be welcoming and friendly.

A person's appearance gives opportunities to make assumptions about their way of life, status, social position, health and self-esteem. A person who appears well groomed is assumed to think well enough of themselves to make the effort to do this. However, appearances can be misleading; for example, someone who is immaculately turned out may have made this effort because they place great significance on what others think of them. Unlike many aspects of non-verbal communication, we can control aspects of our appearance. Dietitians need to consider the appropriateness of what they wear and how they present themselves to the patient group with which they are working (Exercise 8.2). It is easier for the patient to accept the dietitian if the dietitian's appearance is appropriate to her role and fits the patient's expectations. Many different aspects beside appearance are used in forming first impressions, some of which are listed here (see Exercise 8.3):

- Age
- Gender
- Attitudes
- Intelligence
- Attractiveness (hairstyle, skin tone, eyes, teeth)
- Opinions
- Personality
- Character
- Physique – weight, height, posture
- Cultural background
- Possible occupation
- Education
- Temperament
- Financial status
- Voice.

The importance of any particular aspect varies from person to person and according to the situation; for example, attractiveness may be most important at a party, whereas education and attitude may be more important at a job interview.

Exercise 8.2

Think about the effect of the 'white coat', the hallmark of a dietitian's professional status in the hospital environment. If you wear one, how do you do this – casually or formally? Whether or not you wear a white coat, does your appearance represent who you are? Do you feel comfortable with it? Have you been through your wardrobe recently? Do you throw away or give away clothes you no longer wear or which no longer fit your image, or do you hang on to them?

Exercise 8.3

Think of a recent interview you have conducted with a new patient. When forming your first impression, which aspects of the patient were important to you? What aspects can you recall? What assumptions did you make about this person?

First impressions are useful in predicting the behaviour of the other person and deciding on the way to behave in response. However, there are drawbacks. We may be influenced too much by one particular aspect, for example attractiveness. When we attribute someone with many of the characteristics of a particular type we treat them as a stereotype. This leads us to expect people to behave in the same way each time.

We also assign a status to the other person and to ourselves (Exercise 8.4). If we place someone in a higher status than ourselves we may feel nervous. If we place someone in a lower status than ourselves we may patronise them. We are likely to treat the predictions and assumptions we make as facts, forgetting that each person is a unique individual and therefore different from another.

Exercise 8.4

In your interactions in the next 24 hours be aware of the status you assign to the other person and to yourself. In what way do you think this affects your communication with that person?

Once formed, first impressions are difficult to change. Further information is used to reinforce our first impression and we tend to dismiss any which is not consistent with this. As we become more aware of the way in which we categorise people and the errors that may arise from doing this, we become more able to accept others as they are rather than as we expect them to be. We can amend our concept of someone and add to it as we go along by keeping an open mind and assessing impressions continually. Letting go of first impressions allows us to relate with others moment to moment instead of relating to our idea of how we think they should be.

While the dietitian is forming a first impression of her patient, they are forming a first impression of her. A dietitian wanting to show a friendly attitude can do so by:

- adopting an open posture with uncrossed arms and legs;
- speaking in a soft tone of voice;
- smiling;
- making eye contact;
- leaning towards the other person;
- shaking hands.

We find it easier to accept a first impression if it is appropriate to the situation and meets our expectations. The impression we generally take away with us is an overall one based on several characteristics rather than on one in particular. However, if one aspect strikes us as out of place, for example appearance, then this is what will stay in our minds. This is true of both patient and dietitian. Having paid attention to the physical framework and focused on preparing mentally for the interview, the dietitian needs to pay attention to specific tasks which make up the structural framework. Some of these will be familiar, for example taking a diet history. Less familiar may be processes such as contracting and monitoring the relationship. The way in which the dietitian communicates throughout plays a crucial part. The first task concerns opening the interview.

Opening the interview

This stage sets the tone for what follows. Therefore how we meet, greet and introduce ourselves plays a significant part in our first impression as described above and is further discussed in relation to transcultural communication in Chapter 11. The talk at the beginning of the interview usually involves social niceties or 'safe talk'. This includes introductions, showing someone to their seat or enquiring about their appointment. In social situations we use phrases such as 'How do you do?' as a way of greeting. We often ask 'How are you?' not really expecting the other person to expound about their health but to reply 'I'm all right', 'Fine', 'OK' or something similar. When those involved do not make introductions clearly and confidently the communications which follow are more strained. The customary way of making introductions varies in different cultures and this is further explored in Chapter 11.

Exercise 8.5

In the interview situation, what are the ways you introduce yourself and greet your patient? How do you feel when doing this? What information are you assimilating during this safe talk period?

While getting seated, making the introductions and establishing how each of you want to be addressed both dietitian and patient will be forming their first impressions of each other. Usually the dietitian then is the one to initiate conversation. The starting point for a first meeting is likely to be the doctor's referral or the previous time the patient saw the dietitian. For a follow-up appointment the starting point is likely to be what has occurred for the patient since their last visit. The following are some suggestions:

- 'How can I help you?'
- 'I'm wondering how you feel about seeing a dietitian?'
- 'I'm wondering if this is the first time you've been to see a dietitian?'
- 'I'm wondering what was your reaction when the doctor suggested that you see a dietitian?'
- 'How have you been since we last met?'

These opening statements or questions are ways of inviting the patient to talk. As she listens the dietitian will be forming an idea about the patient's motivation.

The interview is now progressing to the middle stage.

Exercise 8.6

The following are four ways in which a patient replies to a dietitian's enquiry:

- 'The doctor said I should come to see you.'
- 'I've been waiting for an appointment to see you for a long time.'
- 'I saw a dietitian years ago but I can't remember much about it.'
- 'I've not been feeling too good since I last saw you.'

Imagine yourself listening to each of these remarks. What are your thoughts and how would you respond to each.

Middles

Setting the agenda

This important feature can easily be missed out because it has either not been considered or not made explicit. As a result the agenda of both patient and dietitian can remain hidden. Setting an agenda defines the interview and makes its purpose clear. It is also a valuable opportunity to establish boundaries relating to time limits and confidentiality. This is also the time to establish the reason for the patient's referral and the expectations the patient has. It could also be an appropriate time to explain how a change in diet can help the patient. Here are three ways of setting agendas, each one reflecting a different attitude and role of the dietitian.

DIETITIAN: (*to a patient*) We have 20 minutes in which to discuss your diet. What I'd like to do is first to weigh you and then go through what you usually have to eat to see if there are any alterations that need to be made.

In the above example the dietitian establishes herself as the one in control. In the following example the dietitian invites the patient to set the agenda, reflecting an open approach which allows the patient to take control.

DIETITIAN: (*to a patient*) How can I help you? We have 20 minutes in which to talk and if we need longer we can arrange to meet again another time.

A third option is to set the agenda together, which some dietitians may consider more appropriate at a follow-up appointment. In the following example the dietitian is including both herself and the patient and establishing a relationship in which she is willing for the control to be shared.

DIETITIAN: We have 20 minutes in which to talk and if we need longer we can arrange to meet again another time. Is there any particular aspect of your diet you would like to talk about? (*waits for answer*)
PATIENT: Well . . . I'm wondering how I can keep to my diet when the rest of the family want different things to eat.
DIETITIAN: (*responds by reflecting*) You would like to discuss how you can fit your diet in with the family. I'd like to go through your diet with you to get an idea of what you usually eat, (*stating her agenda*) so shall we begin by you telling me what you and the family usually have and then we can see how this fits in for with your diet? (*making a suggestion*).

Exercise 8.7

Imagine yourself conducting an interview with a patient. You have been asked to assess the diet of an overweight, middle-aged business man with abnormal liver function tests, suggesting he has a high alcohol intake. What would be your agenda? How would you establish this with the patient? What boundaries would you establish and how would you do this? How would you demonstrate your understanding of the patient's presenting concerns?

Sometimes the dietitian may find it is necessary to set her agenda completely on one side because the patient's needs are so obviously not concerned with diet. This occurs in the example illustrated in the next two sections in which the patient is concerned about her daughter's marriage crisis. In such a situation the dietitian focuses on applying her counselling skills while being aware of her boundaries concerning time, role and confidentiality. She is also assessing her patient's motivation to change her diet.

Assessing motivation

A patient's motivation to change their eating behaviour will fluctuate from time to time so that an assessment made at the initial meeting may be different from that made at a later date. The patient's self-assessment and the assessment of the dietitian may be the same or different. When the patient's motivation is at a low ebb the dietitian may think 'How can I motivate this person?' or 'What will motivate this person?'. She is likely to give advice and instruction (Chapter 1). Her tactics are likely to be persuasion and her method of communication likely to be manipulation. On the other hand she may wonder 'How motivated is this person?' and 'What is holding this person back from changing their diet?'. She is then more likely to attempt to understand the patient from their frame of reference and will be endeavouring to demonstrate a person-centred approach. If she judges the relationship between her and the patient to be secure enough, she may decide it is appropriate to ask the patient these questions directly. However, if she thinks to do so might jeopardise the helping relationship she is fostering, she may decide to express herself less inquisitively and more tentatively, for example by saying, 'I'm wondering what you think is holding you back from making (or maintaining) these changes in your diet.' The way in which the dietitian expresses herself can make the difference between aiding or disabling the helping process (Chapter 6) and encouraging or discouraging motivation in the patient.

In assessing motivation many dietitians find it helpful to have in mind the framework for the phases of change (Prochaska & DiClemente 1986) described in Chapter 4. The following example illustrates how a dietitian might apply this.

> PATIENT: (*abruptly*) The doctor said I should come to see you but it's really a waste of your time.
>
> DIETITIAN: (*assesses the patient is in the first phase, i.e. 'not interested in making changes'. Decides to acknowledge this knowing that doing so is likely to lead to an exploration of other issues in the patient's life. She speaks calmly*) You don't understand why the doctor thinks it important that you make changes to your diet? Or is it that you know what changes to make but have been finding it difficult to put them into practice?
>
> PATIENT: (*impatiently*) Oh I know the doctor thinks I need to lose weight for my blood pressure. I've been on diets on and off for years. I know what I should do but going on a diet right now is just about the last thing I need!

DIETITIAN: (*registers the remark about a long struggle to lose weight, decides to respond to the stress implied in what has been said*) Changing your diet now would be adding to your stress?

PATIENT: Absolutely! I've got enough on my plate coping with the grandchildren. Just when I thought I could have a bit of time for myself my daughter leaves her husband and she and the kids land on my doorstep. (*bursts into tears*).

Thinking about what the patient has said and what she has expressed through her non-verbal communication the dietitian realises that this interaction has reinforced her assessment that her patient is not ready to make dietary changes at the present time. Many times, however, there is an incongruity between the verbal and the non-verbal communication so that the dietitian is not sure about her assessment. This is valuable to observe as it most probably reflects the patient's ambivalence about changing their diet.

In the example described above the dietitian realises she now has several choices in the way she responds to what the patient has just said. She can either respond to the detail (the breakdown of the daughter's marriage) thus inviting the patient to expand on this (which is very likely to lead them into non-diet related areas beyond the role of the dietitian) or adopt an authoritative role (see 'Continuum of control' in Chapter 1) by drawing a line under what the patient has said and deliberately focusing on the patient's diet; alternatively she can focus on another aspect of the interview framework which is making a contract as described in the next section.

Making a contract

Continuing the above interview the dietitian decides to make her patient's present distress the priority. At the same time she realises she has limited time left for the interview and her responsibility as a dietitian is both to her patient and to the doctor who referred the patient as well as to the other patients she has yet to see.

DIETITIAN: (*moves the tissues to within reach of the patient, focuses on the patient's distress and says gently*) Help yourself to tissues if you want some. (*summarising the patient's last remarks*) You are finding you have a lot to cope with at the moment.

PATIENT: Yes . . . too much . . . but I don't want to bother you. It's just that I can't see how I can follow a diet when it is all so chaotic at home. My daughter hardly eats a thing and the children want different things all the time. . . . I haven't got time to think of me.

DIETITIAN: (*paraphrasing*) From what you're saying now doesn't seem a good time to change your diet when you and your family are already coping with big changes. (*sharing what is in her mind*) I'm wondering if your doctor knows how you feel about changing your diet when you have these problems at home?

PATIENT: No . . . there wasn't time. . . . He's given me some pills to take for my blood pressure and he wants to see me in two weeks. Do you think I should tell him?

DIETITIAN: (*states her position*) The doctor will expect me to let him know I have discussed your diet with you. I can say that you came to see me, you were feeling very stressed due to a change in family circumstances and did not feel able to make major changes to your diet at the moment. (*puts options for action*) Then you can decide when you next see him if you want to tell him about it. Or if you want me to I can give him the details. Which would you prefer?

PATIENT: (*sounding relieved*) Oh I like the first idea. Then I can decide because things may have changed when I next see him. Do I come and see you again?

DIETITIAN: (*invites the patient to choose*) Would you like to?

PATIENT: Perhaps when things have settled down at home and I can think about my diet. It's just so difficult at the moment. I feel better having told you a bit about it. I know we have to get things sorted. My daughter is seeing a solicitor this week. It's early days but we'll get through it somehow.

DIETITIAN: (*clarifying the patient's preferred option*) So would you like me to ask the doctor to refer you again when you want some help with your diet?

PATIENT: Yes please and thank you for your help.

In the process of contracting with the patient the dietitian has:

- summarised what has been said so far;
- accurately identified the patient's presenting concerns;
- formulated and discussed goals or the course of action;
- handled questions;
- made arrangements about a further meeting.

When a patient has a greater motivation to change their diet than in the example above, the task of making a contract is likely to come at a later stage, for example after a discussion about diet.

Taking a diet history

Asking a patient what they usually eat and investigating the frequency of food consumption is a very familiar part of the dietetic interview. Although it is convenient in many ways to use the standard format of starting at the beginning of the day and working logically through each mealtime, checking amounts, portion sizes and preparation of dishes, it does presume that all patients will fit into this pattern. The dietitian is likely to phrase her remarks to encourage the patient to conform with what is expected. The following is an example from an interview which demonstrates this.

> DIETITIAN: First of all I need to know what you usually have to eat. What did you have for breakfast yesterday for example?
> PATIENT: Oh, just a bowl of cereal. Nothing much.
> DIETITIAN: Nothing else? What do you have for lunch?
> PATIENT: Yesterday I had bread and cheese.
> DIETITIAN: Do you usually have that?
> PATIENT: No, not always. It depends. Sometimes I have a sandwich or soup. Something like that.
> DIETITIAN: And in the evening. What did you have for your main meal?
> PATIENT: Mm . . . let me see . . . a pizza. That's what I had yesterday.

In practice additional questions concerning the type of cereal the patient eats, whether they take sugar and the amount of milk used, are likely to be asked. If we examine the interactions we notice that the dietitian has set her agenda at the beginning and established herself as the one in charge by saying what she needs from the interview. She follows this with a question which reinforces this. The patient adopts the position of someone who is being interrogated. A series of direct questions follows (Chapter 7) and short replies which offer little apart from the information directly asked for. In the following extract reflective responding is used (Chapter 6).

> DIETITIAN: I'd like you to tell me about the food you usually eat. You might find the easiest way is to recall what you had yesterday.
> PATIENT: Yesterday . . . let me see now . . . mm . . . oh yes I had a pizza.
> DIETITIAN: A pizza.
> PATIENT: Yes . . . and garlic bread. And a bottle of wine. You see I went out with some friends in the evening. It was someone's birthday.
> DIETITIAN: So yesterday you went out for a pizza in the evening as you were celebrating someone's birthday.
> PATIENT: Yes. I had that quite late – about 9. Usually I eat about 7, as soon as I get in from work. I'm really hungry by then as I only have a sandwich at lunch time.
> DIETITIAN: You normally have a sandwich for lunch and your evening meal at about 7.
> PATIENT: Yes – and I always have breakfast. Cereal and toast you know. . . .
> DIETITIAN: So your usual pattern is to have cereal and toast for breakfast, a sandwich for lunch and your main meal in the evening.

In this interview the dietitian again focuses on the agenda at the beginning but this time includes the patient ('I would like you to tell me about the food you usually have to eat'). She invites the patient to take charge ('You might find the easiest way is to recall what you had yesterday'). The patient initially replies in the same way as in the previous extract, but instead of questioning the patient, the dietitian responds by reflecting a key word ('pizza') which the patient has said.

The dietitian responds by paraphrasing and summarising content or meaning (Chapter 6). This results in the patient replying more fully and the dietitian gaining more information, e.g. yesterday being unusual (a celebration evening meal), the patient's eating habits (hungry when gets in from work) and problem ('I only have a sandwich at lunch time'). At this point the dietitian has a choice: to reflect the patient's hunger or to focus on the topic in hand (taking a diet history). She chooses the latter and summarises the meals described so far ('You normally have a sandwich for lunch and your evening meal at about 7'). The patient then completes the inventory by talking about breakfast and the dietitian concludes by summarising the meal pattern.

In recent times meal patterns for many people have become less structured. Snacking throughout the day seems to be more common and it is probably more difficult for patients who do this to recall what they have eaten. The dietitian who uses reflective responding rather than direct questioning to encourage her patient to remember what they have eaten is, arguably, more likely to obtain accurate information. However, others may feel under pressure of time constraints and decide to ask a series of direct closed questions about food intake. They trust that their relationship with the patient is sufficiently well established by the time they come to take a dietary history that this method will not hinder the helping process. However, when taking a diet history is led by the dietitian she will not know what additional information may have been disclosed if instead this had been led by the patient.

Dietitians who are familiar with asking short, direct questions in order to obtain specific information as quickly as possible in a structured format, may consider that accuracy of information is sacrificed when not using this approach. On the other hand asking a lot of direct questions risks damaging the communication (Bolton 1986), as patients who feel interrogated are more likely to give answers they think are expected rather than an honest reply.

Exercise 8.8

When you next take a diet history focus your attention on the questions you ask and the remarks you make. Look for occasions when you ask leading questions or expect a particular response. You may want to record yourself taking a diet history so that you can play it back and listen closely. (Be sure to ask the patient if this is alright with them, explaining to them that you are doing it for your professional development.)

Giving dietary advice

Dietitians have become more aware in recent years of the impact of professionally presented leaflets and diet sheets. These are usually used as a substitute for the spoken word or to reinforce what has been discussed. The image that dietitians present is reflected in the written material they use. Through the spoken and written word the dietitian aims to help people modify their diets. She makes suggestions for improvement, explains to patients what they can eat without restriction, what they must avoid eating and what they can eat in moderation. She suggests, advises, informs and instructs. She does this through direct consultations and written material. Referring to the continuum of control described in Chapter 1, these methods demonstrate the dietitian's authority. When communicating in these ways, it is important that she is aware of the pitfalls described below.

Lecturing

One of the main ways in which dietitians gain information themselves is by attending lectures. Qualified dietitians are expected to give lectures to student nurses and others. Lecturing is therefore a familiar way of giving and receiving information. It is hardly surprising therefore that dietitians, often without realising it, give their patients mini-lectures. Although lecturing is one way to give a lot of information to a large number of people in a short space of time, it is not an effective way to facilitate learning on an individual basis. When being lectured the listener is not involved and so may feel 'talked at' rather than 'talked to'. Concentration span is quickly exceeded. Once this happens the listener feels overwhelmed and confused and stops listening.

When the dietitian is fully involved in giving information she is unlikely to notice her patient's non-verbal signals. If she were to notice she might interpret these as a sign that she should repeat or re-emphasise her point. In this way she is encouraged to continue with her 'lecture'. She has much knowledge herself and wants to fully inform her patient. She does not want to be guilty of omitting anything which could jeopardise the patient's health. In her efforts to ensure she fulfils her obligation to inform her patient, she may overlook the fact that the patient is not understanding and has stopped listening.

Jargon

Another pitfall is using scientific language when talking to a patient. Dietitians accumulate a vast amount of professional language, as do all professions. Some of this becomes familiar to those outside the profession and is incorporated into everyday vocabulary. For example many terms specific to the computer industry are used nowadays in a general context. Although 'calories' is a term used in everyday language, it is doubtful if many of those using it know what it means technically. Similarly, metric units of measurement used by dietitians may not be understood by the patient. Although dietitians may realise this, they may not always be aware of when they slip into such language. Mirroring the language used by the patient is a way in which the dietitian can ensure she is using language which her patient understands (Chapter 6).

Using 'we' and 'I'

By using simple words such as 'we' rather than 'I' dietitians can set themselves apart from the patient and add power to their position. The collective 'we' implies the backing of all dietitians. It can also imply the agreement of the medical profession and so carry great weight. The effect on the patient is that they feel outnumbered and overpowered by a large authoritative body. The following is an example of using the collective 'we':

PATIENT: How much can I have?
DIETITIAN: A small amount would be all right. We don't want you to do without altogether but you need to restrict the amount you have. As the doctor said, your blood levels are on the high side and we know that people who eat too much fat are at greater risk.

Here the dietitian is using the collective 'we' to effectively distance herself from the patient. This is probably not what she intends. She may want to add weight to her point of view if she is unsure of her ground or if she thinks the information is not what the patient wants to hear. By using the collective 'we' the dietitian identifies herself as a member of a larger group. In doing so she reassures herself but separates herself from her patient, which contradicts any previous attempts to create rapport. On hearing the collective 'we' the patient is likely to feel confused thinking that the dietitian who appeared friendly and helpful now seems cooler and more distant. The following example shows this in practice.

PATIENT: That's helpful what you've said but when I get in from work I'm really hungry.
DIETITIAN: You could have more to eat for lunch. We have evidence that regular meals help people to stop nibbling.
PATIENT: *(keeps silent)*

When the dietitian uses reflective responding the effect changes as shown here.

> PATIENT: That's helpful what you've said but when I get in from work I'm really hungry.
> DIETITIAN: By the time you get home you're very hungry.
> PATIENT: Yes, very. It's a long time since lunch. Maybe I ought to have more then or a snack during the afternoon.

Using reflective responding the dietitian has acknowledged the patient's problem, and the patient feels understood and so is encouraged to come up with ideas of his own. The relationship between patient and dietitian is built on co-operation rather than on the position of an expert giving advice to someone who is ignorant.

Risky responses

Failure to make desired changes in eating behaviour is often ascribed, by both patient and dietitian, to lack of willpower on the part of the patient. The dietitian may encourage, admonish, reassure or challenge the patient in order to achieve compliance. Certain responses carry a greater risk than others of blocking further communication and creating defensive behaviour on the part of the patient (Chapter 5). Suggesting, advising, informing and instructing carry a considerable risk of being authoritative rather than facilitative. As a result the patient is likely to make changes to please the dietitian or doctor, rather than feeling empowered to do so for their own well-being.

The patient who follows the dietitian's suggestions and instructions because they have been told to do so, is likely to feel fearful of incurring the dietitian's disapproval or hopeful of receiving her approval at their next visit. The patient may protect themselves from disapproval and disappointment by saying something such as 'I know I haven't done very well. I expect you'll tell me off.' The dietitian is effectively disarmed and is likely to respond by reassuring the patient. Communication is indirect and ultimately dissatisfying to both.

Patients may also invite the dietitian to take responsibility for solving their problems. Remarks such as 'But what can I do?' and 'I know you'll be able to tell me what I should do', are examples. The dietitian responds by giving suggestions and advice and may find that there is no further difficulty. On the other hand the patient may respond with remarks such as, 'I've tried that and it didn't work' and 'I thought you could sort me out'. The dietitian then comes up with different ideas only to find these meet with similar responses. An alternative is for the dietitian to apply a person-centred approach as shown in the example below.

> DIETITIAN: Your blood tests show you have a raised level of cholesterol. Changing your diet may help to bring this down. How do you feel about doing this?
> PATIENT: Well, I'll give it a go if you think it will help.
> DIETITIAN: (*reflecting*) You'll change your diet if this is going to help your health?
> PATIENT: Yes, but does it mean cutting out a lot?
> DIETITIAN: (*giving information*) It means being careful about the amount and type of fat in your diet.
> PATIENT: Oh I don't eat much fat – my wife sees to that. Can I have a list of what I mustn't have, to give to her?
> DIETITIAN: (*meeting patient's request*) This leaflet shows you foods which contain a lot of fat as well as those which do not contain any. It also explains which ones to eat in moderate amounts.
> PATIENT: Thank you. (*takes leaflet and glances at it*) There seems a lot here. Can't you just tell me what I should do?
> DIETITIAN: (*reflecting*) It's a lot to take in at a glance . . . I think it will become clearer if we go through it together.

Exercise 8.9

What is your response to reading the example above? How does this differ from your standard way of giving dietary advice?

Monitoring the relationship

The effect of using reflective responding shows most clearly in the nature of the relationship that is being established. By using reflective responding the dietitian does not imply her own judgements and this allows the patient to reply more openly and explain their diet in a way that makes sense to them. A relationship is formed in which co-operation can occur.

Although this may seem more demanding of the dietitian, the relationship with the patient is more likely to be one in which the patient feels valued and respected and encouraged to talk openly and honestly. This is something for the dietitian to be aware of throughout the interview. By monitoring the relationship the dietitian will be more aware of issues, such as dependency and transference (Chapter 3), and so more able to manage these before they inhibit the work in progress.

The following extract is an example of when the dietitian recognises that her patient is becoming overly dependent on her.

> PATIENT: I don't know how I'll manage when I'm no longer able to come and see you. You keep me on the right track.
>
> DIETITIAN: (*lightly acknowledges appreciation*) Thank you. I'm glad you have found our sessions helpful. (*shares her concern*) I'm a bit concerned though when I hear you say you don't know how you'll manage without these appointments. (*questions reality of her patient's thinking*) Is that what you really think?
>
> PATIENT: Well I suppose I'll cope but it won't be the same without you to tell me off when I've gained weight. (*gives a small laugh*).
>
> DIETITIAN: (*reflecting key words*) Tell you off! (*drawing on previous work*) As we've discussed before I think you're quick to do that yourself! (*both laugh and dietitian has a sense that the relationship has shifted to being more equal*).
>
> PATIENT: Yes I know. But it won't be the same on my own.
>
> DIETITIAN: (*acknowledges reality in patient's remark*) No it won't be the same. Maybe there are other ways you could get some support so you don't feel so alone?

In asking this last question the dietitian opens up the possibility for the patient to gain a different perspective on her situation. In other words she is inviting her patient to work at Stage 2 of the helping process (Egan 2004).

Tracking the helping process

Using Egan's model can be helpful when monitoring the relationship. As described in Chapter 4, the helping process (Egan 2004) can be broken down into three stages:

- Stage 1 – listening to the patient's story and identifying the problem(s)
- Stage 2 – clarifying what the patient wants
- Stage 3 – ways to achieve goals.

The dietitian who has these stages in mind as the interview progresses is able to track where she and her patient are in this process. This can help her manage her anxiety about having insufficient time.

Many dietitians feel stressed when they need to give the patient information but the patient seems unable to listen. This can result in the dietitian repeating advice, focusing on solving problems, setting goals and planning strategies before the patient is ready to engage with this. From the patient's perspective he may think he has not been fully understood or had enough time to tell the dietitian about his circumstances. The dietitian is working at Stage 3 and the patient is at Stage 1 in the helping process. When the dietitian identifies this and concentrates on using her skills of active listening and reflective responding to help her focus on the patient's needs she will discover that the outcome becomes more satisfying to both. She will then be able to tailor her dietary advice more accurately and the patient will experience being more accepted and respected. As a result the patient will be more able to assimilate the dietary advice given. In other words the patient will be more ready to work at Stage 3 of the helping process when the dietitian has been able to work with him through Stages 1 and 2.

Endings

Closing the interview

The reader is advised to read this section in conjunction with the sections on 'When, how and where to refer' and 'How to end' in Chapter 4. Closing the interview will take a matter of minutes when the interview that has taken place is the only meeting. However, if patient and dietitian have been meeting for a series of appointments the dietitian will need longer to prepare for ending, for example one if not two meetings.

Acknowledging the ending

Acknowledging the closing of each interview is the responsibility of the dietitian. She needs to find a way of remarking that it is time to draw the interview to a close. For example she may say 'I'm aware we need to finish in five minutes' or 'Time is running out for us – we will need to stop in a few minutes.' Although the number of appointments will have been discussed at the contracting stage it is important that the dietitian refers to the fact that their work together is coming to an end **before** the last appointment rather than assume that the patient recalls this. In addition it is helpful to acknowledge at the penultimate appointment that they have one more planned and to acknowledge at the start of the last meeting that this is their last appointment.

People react in different ways to an ending. Some will feel a need to hurry up, to get in as much as possible in the time remaining and may elaborate on what they have already said or even broach new topics; others may stop abruptly as though they need to leave immediately.

Inviting a patient to talk about their reaction can lead to helpful disclosures. For example a dietitian could say 'I'm wondering if you think you've had enough time or whether you need more?' or 'I'm not sure if you feel relieved or maybe anxious about this being our last appointment? A patient may then share concerns about managing without the support of the dietitian in which case the dietitian needs to allow time to explore these concerns with her patient.

Summarising what has taken place

This fulfils the function of clarifying and reinforcing what their work together has been about and it is particularly valuable for the patient if they can do this for themselves. The dietitian can encourage the patient by asking what they have found helpful, what they will be putting into practice, what difficulties they think they will find in the future. These questions are likely to yield information and further questions for discussion so the dietitian needs to allow adequate time for this to occur. If the patient finds self-acknowledgement too difficult the dietitian can summarise what she thinks the patient has learned from their work together and this provides encouragement and affirmation for the patient. Giving this in a way that is not patronising requires the dietitian to examine her attitude to her patient, her ability to be honest and genuine in sharing her thoughts and her skill in focusing on specific behaviour (Chapters 6, 14 and 15).

What next?

In helping the patient to clarify how they will manage in the future the dietitian may want to refer to previous discussions about resources and support available. She may want to discuss other sources of professional help and the reader is recommended to read the guidelines in the section on referral in Chapter 4. When clarifying what she herself or her dietetic department can offer by way of ongoing support she needs to give detailed information about how the patient can make contact in the future. This stage is important for the patient to feel supported. It also confirms for the dietitian and the patient that their work together is drawing to a close. This can be particularly difficult for the dietitian who undervalues the help she has given and for the patient whose needs have not been met. Both will feel pressure to make further appointments. The dietitian needs to be aware of her own motives when offering a follow-up appointment. The following questions are useful to consider:

- How practical is a further appointment for the patient and for myself?
- Will I be seeing the patient or is it likely to be another dietitian? Do I explain this to the patient?
- Am I offering this because the patient wants to come back? Or because I do not want to let go?
- How do I offer another appointment? Do I say 'I'd like to see you again' or do I ask 'Would you like to come again?'
- If we agree to another appointment how do we decide when this is to be? Is the patient aware of the system for making/cancelling appointments? Are they reliable or likely to cancel or not attend?
- What will be the purpose of a further appointment? Can this be clarified?

With full caseloads it is more and more important for this process of closure to be managed in a mutually fulfilling way.

Saying goodbye

When a fulfilling helping relationship has been established saying goodbye can be difficult. Neither may want to do this and each may wait for the other to take the lead. Conversely one may want to end it quickly and the other may be left with an unsatisfactory feeling of incompletion. As explained in Chapter 4, endings can arouse intense anxiety especially when the relationship established has been of some depth and meaning to each person. In a dietetic context termination of a working contract with a patient cannot always be planned and there may be no opportunity to complete their work together. For example a dietitian may have been seeing a terminally ill patient over a considerable period of time and the ending of their appointments may occur because of the patient's death. Frequently the ending may occur due to the discharge from hospital of patients before the dietitian has had a chance to see them. In outpatient settings it is more likely to be because the patient stops attending appointments or the dietitian moves to another area of work. Unsatisfactory endings as well as problematic interviews are times when it is valuable for the dietitian to be able to review her work in a structured way either on her own, with a colleague or with a supervisor/mentor (Chapter 15).

After the interview

When reviewing an interview with a colleague many dietitians find it difficult to stay focused. The colleague may want to know more about

the patient and question the dietitian about the patient's circumstances which raises issues about confidentiality. The dietitian may
want to consider how she can describe her patient accurately while
not revealing identity details, for example not referring to a patient by
name or else using a pseudonym. Dietitian and colleague may recall
other similar cases or find themselves having a generalised discussion
about related issues. When they get sidetracked in this way their time
together is likely to come to a hurried close with both feeling somewhat dissatisfied. Table 8.2 provides a framework to help the dietitian
stay focused when reviewing an interview and is designed to be used
in addition to any data about dietary information.

Table 8.2   Review of a dietetic interview.

Identity details
  Who is my patient? E.g. male/female, age

Health history
  What is their current health like?
  What is their medical history?
  Does the patient appear to have any mental health problems?

Social information
  What is their occupation?
  What is their cultural background?
  Do they live alone/with someone?
  Do they have contact with their family?
  What support do they think they have?

Presenting issues
  What brought them to see me now?
  What do they consider to be a problem?
  What do I consider to be their problem?
  What is the significance of food in the patient's life?

Working together
  What do I think the patient wanted from me?
  What was I able to offer?
  Am I able to provide what the patient wanted?
  In what way do I think I helped the patient?
  How would I describe our relationship?
  How did I feel during the interview?
  How able is the patient to take care of themselves, e.g. to follow guidelines?
  Does the patient need extra resources, e.g. an interpreter or support with a
  disability?

As the dietitian
  What were my concerns?
  What did I find satisfying about this interview(s)?
  What have I learned about myself as a result of my work with this patient?

In thinking through an interview in this way the dietitian can monitor the relationship between herself and the patient and can increase the likelihood of providing a relationship which is helpful to the patient and rewarding for herself.

References

Bolton, R. (1986) *People Skills*. Prentice Hall, Sydney.

Egan, G. (2004) *The Skilled Helper – A Problem Management Approach to Helping*, 7th edn. Thomson Wadsworth, Belmont, CA.

Prochaska, J.O. & DiClemente, C.C. (1986) Towards a comprehensive model of change. In: *Treating Addictive Behaviours: Processes of Change* (eds W.R. Miller & N. Heather). Plenum, New York.

Chapter 9

Loss and Bereavement

'Can I see another's woe
And not be in sorrow too?
Can I see another's grief
And not seek for kind relief?'

William Blake: On another's sorrow

In this chapter I discuss:

- How loss concerns dietitians
- The need to grieve
- How the dietitian can help
- Loss of weight – a loss or a gain?
- Loss of self-esteem
- Loss of health – living under threat of death
- Loss of appetite
- Support for the patient and the dietitian

How loss concerns dietitians

Dietitians frequently encounter patients who are suffering loss of some kind. This chapter aims to help their understanding of the process they are dealing with, both within themselves and their patients, and offers some practical suggestions for them to consider. The subject of loss is not an easy one to reflect on and the reader may feel uncomfortable at times. She may prefer to take her time in reading this chapter, possibly coming back to it at a later date.

Loss and gain are integral parts of any change (Marris 1992) and for a change to take place effectively we need to mourn the losses and acknowledge the gains. Exercise 9.1 is designed to increase the reader's awareness of losses and gains that they have recently experienced.

> **Exercise 9.1**
>
> Think over the past 12 months and write down events that have happened to you, e.g. change of job, moving house. Write these down under one of two headings – gains or losses. For example 'new job' may be a gain. Now write down a loss associated with each gain, for example 'no longer have A as a colleague' could be a loss associated with 'new job'. Similarly with each event in the 'loss' column note a gain. For example, a loss might be 'no longer working in paediatrics' and a gain that has occurred as a result of moving into another field might be 'I am widening my experience'. Be aware of how you feel as you do this exercise. It is useful to do it with a partner so that you can talk about the process. Use the opportunity to practise your skills at active listening.

There are times when the gains associated with a change clearly outweigh the losses. When this happens we think of the change as a desirable one and feel pleasure and satisfaction when we realise the benefits that result. When a change occurs in which the losses outweigh the gains we think of the change as 'bad' and are likely to feel sad, depressed, angry and powerless. In adjusting to loss we go through a process of bereavement and although this is usually associated with death, the bereavement process occurs when adjusting to any loss.

Those in ill-health suffer a loss of their natural healthy state. The loss may be for a short period before health is regained, as in acute illness, or the loss may necessitate an adjustment to living with a chronic condition. Some patients may find their loss particularly difficult to deal with as the change in their health may raise psychological issues as well as practical problems. The following are examples of some of the losses which dietitians are likely to encounter in their patients:

- loss of health and well-being;
- loss of a limb following amputation;
- loss of mobility after a stroke;
- loss of function as a result of disease (e.g. loss of heart function due to coronary heart disease);
- loss of appetite;
- loss of weight.

Other losses may coincide or occur as a result of any of the above. For example, patients may lose their job because of ill health and relationships may break down under the strain of ill health. A patient may feel overwhelmed by the loss of home and family and may suffer considerable loss of self-esteem.

When confronted with another's loss we often feel anxious and unsure about what to say or do. We may want to help the other person, yet be concerned lest what we say results in them becoming more upset. We may fear becoming upset ourselves. In the face of our own anxiety and the other person's distress, we often give reassurance in the hope that we will both then feel better. As shown in Chapter 6, the way in which we give reassurance can carry a considerable risk of creating a barrier in the relationship between two people.

The need to grieve

Grieving is a necessary and natural process that we undergo when we suffer a loss. We feel a sense of loss when the attachment we have formed for someone or something is broken. Psychiatrist John Bowlby (1997, 1998, 2004) has written extensively on the subject of attachment and loss. Loss arouses intense anxiety. Grieving is about resolving the conflicts between wanting things to be as they were before the loss occurred and wanting to move forward to continue with our lives. We have a compulsion to preserve the continuity in our lives (Marris 1992), and when a change occurs we suffer a break in this continuity. During the period of grieving we struggle to make sense of our loss, to give it meaning and to regain our sense of continuity. In order for this internal process to take place we need:

- to be cared for, e.g. to have food provided;
- to talk about the loss;
- to have someone to listen;
- to have time alone;
- to be accepted the way we are and not to feel that others disapprove.

Identifying and expressing feelings is one of the tasks of grieving (Worden 2003), and in offering a patient the opportunity to talk about their loss the dietitian is demonstrating her willingness to help. In the way she listens and responds, the dietitian can make a significant contribution to a patient's healing process.

Culturally it is often not acceptable to show our grief openly and so we may deny it or try to hide it. When denial and suppression are prolonged, we suffer long-term emotional pain and stress. Those in the caring professions who can recognise grief and can support, rather than reassure, someone through the period of adapting to loss (mourning) are providing skilled and needed help.

Our reactions to grief

We become attached to people, places and objects of all kinds and the more significant the attachment the greater our sense of loss when this is broken. Our reactions to loss are individual and unique. We experience a profusion of feelings and physical sensations. Confusion is one of the major sources of stress accompanying a bereavement. We may behave in irrational and atypical ways that alarm us and those around us, and we may experience a loss of control. Our reactions may be immediate or they may be delayed depending upon the level of shock we experience.

Exercise 9.2 is designed to increase the reader's awareness of her own thoughts, feelings and actions in response to a loss.

Exercise 9.2

Take a sheet of paper and divide it into three sections. Head one section 'Feelings', another 'Thoughts' and the third 'Behaviour'. Now think of something you have recently mislaid or lost, such as a book. List your thoughts and feelings and the actions you took at the time. For example:

Feeling	*Thought*	*Behaviour*
Puzzled	'Where's it gone?'	Search room
Anxious	'I can't find it'	Search more frantically
Annoyed	'Who's taken it?'	Accuse colleague
Sad	'I've lost it'	Eyes fill with tears
Miserable	'I'll never get it back'	Sit with head in hands

The process of grieving

Elizabeth Kubler-Ross (2005) in her work with the dying, identified a pattern of denial, anger, bargaining and depression experienced by those who are bereaved, before they reach an acceptance of their loss. Someone who has at first denied the loss (e.g. 'It's not true') will experience times of intense anger (e.g. 'It's all the doctor's fault') and will make bargains in an attempt to redress the loss (e.g. 'If I try really hard from now on it will be all right'). In the next moment they may deny again that the loss has occurred (e.g. 'I just don't believe it').

Dietitians supporting someone through a loss need to remember that this is a normal process. The bereaved person is likely to feel confused and may indicate that they think they are going mad, such is the welter of thoughts and feelings they suffer. It can be helpful to be told that such thoughts are normal and acceptable. People suffering loss who are told to 'snap out of it' or 'pull themselves together' are hindered in their grieving and may be prevented from working through the process. Those who have not been allowed to complete their grieving and who get stuck in the process suffer long-term physical and emotional distress. The process of grieving is one of considerable stress and disturbances in sleep patterns and eating behaviour, and misuse of drugs and alcohol may occur.

How the dietitian can help

A dietitian who has an understanding of bereavement, an ability to recognise the different aspects of the process and the necessary skills in listening can provide invaluable help to a patient who is grieving. A dietitian can learn to:

- recognise various reactions to grief;
- provide the core conditions of empathy, acceptance and genuineness;
- listen actively (attending, reflective responding);
- provide practical care as appropriate;
- offer practical information about professional support, e.g. national or local branch of Cruse (see Appendix 2).

Here are some tips which will support someone who is bereaved (adapted from information from Cruse Bereavement Care):

- Let your genuine concern and care show.
- Be available to listen or to help with whatever seems needed at the time.
- Say you are sorry about what has happened and that they are suffering pain.
- Allow them to express as much unhappiness as they want to share.
- Encourage them to be patient and not expect too much of themselves.
- Allow them to talk about their loss as much and as often as they want to. They won't have forgotten their loss so there is no need to avoid mentioning it.
- Talk about the special endearing qualities of what they have lost.
- Let them know that they have done everything they could.

A dietitian may feel helpless when faced with a patient's distress and may tell herself that she cannot help. This thought may stop her reaching out and her discomfort may mean she avoids talking about the patient's loss. For the patient who is bereaved, the avoidance adds pain to an already painful experience. In an effort to be helpful the dietitian may say that she understands how the patient feels. This is likely to produce an angry response as shown in the following example.

> PATIENT: (*talking about recent death of husband*) I just can't be bothered to cook for myself. It was different when he was alive; I had a reason to do it then. Nowadays I'm just not hungry.
> DIETITIAN: (*in a sympathetic tone of voice*) I know how you feel.
> PATIENT: (*angrily*) How can you know – you're not me. You can't possibly understand.

The dietitian can demonstrate her empathy more effectively by reflecting, as shown here.

> PATIENT: (*talking about recent death of husband*) I just can't be bothered to cook for myself. It was different when he was alive; I had a reason to do it then. Nowadays I'm just not hungry.
> DIETITIAN: Since your husband died you feel it's all too much effort to cook for yourself, especially when you have no appetite.
> PATIENT: Yes, that's it. I'm worried about my weight – I've lost a lot since Bill went.

Those who are bereaved do not want to be judged, told what they should do or how they should feel. The following remarks are typical of ones that are well meant but unhelpful.

'You ought to be feeling better by now.'
'In time you can always have another. . . .'
'Just think of all the things you have. . . .'
'It doesn't do to dwell on it.'
'Just put it all behind you now and get on with life.'
'Perhaps if you had/hadn't done. . . .'
'At least you've got. . . .'

Loss of weight – a loss or a gain?

Helping someone to lose excess weight forms a large part of the work of most dietitians. Weight loss, when perceived as desirable, is thought of as something to be gained. Achieving the target weight is seen as a goal to aim for and is often used as a means of encouraging the patient. Both patient and dietitian may discount the existence of the losses and may focus on the gains associated with a reduction in weight. Acknowledging the losses helps the patient feel understood, supported and more motivated to follow the dietary advice.

Some losses associated with a reduction in weight are more obvious and easier to talk about than others, for example the loss of a wardrobe as clothes which have been comfortable no longer fit. Less clear and more difficult to talk about is the loss of identity and security the patient may feel as her body becomes less familiar. Anxiety associated with loss may lead a patient to eat more. Changes in body weight may involve a psychologically demanding change in self-image. Issues concerning the patient's relationship to food, herself and other people can evoke intense anxiety and psychological pain, resulting in internal conflict and ambivalence about following dietary advice. Working with those in eating distress is covered more fully in the section on eating disorders in Chapter 12. The dietitian who is aware that underlying issues are likely to contribute to her patient's inability to lose weight is in a position to be more empathic. She may want to offer information about other sources of help (Chapter 4).

In helping a patient to explore their concerns, the dietitian may find herself examining her own relationship to food and her body. Her own difficulties may make it hard for her to offer her patient the core conditions of empathy, acceptance and genuineness. Awareness of her difficulties may lead her to consider professional help for herself (Chapter 15).

Loss of self-esteem

When we lose something or someone to whom we have been attached, we may feel cut adrift and uncertain. A sense of loss of direction may accompany feelings of worthlessness and inadequacy. The patient who has lost self-confidence is likely to seek reassurance in a number of ways, such as:

- 'You do think I'm doing all right, don't you?'
- 'I'm not taking up too much of your time, am I?'
- 'I don't want to be a nuisance.'
- 'I'm not really worth bothering with.'
- 'You've got better things to do than see me.'

It is not easy to respond to these remarks except by agreeing or denying what has been said. The dietitian may give the expected answer because she thinks not to do so would be hurtful, yet in assuring the patient she is not a nuisance, is not taking up too much time and so on, the dietitian may feel irritated, resentful or annoyed. There are various ways in which the dietitian can respond, which affirm the patient's self-worth instead of reinforcing their low self-esteem. Each of the following examples relates to the corresponding remark above:

- 'I think you are coping with a difficult time in the way you know best.'
- 'We have 20 minutes together and if you would like more time we can arrange that.'
- 'I want to help you in whatever way I can.'
- 'I think you are undervaluing yourself.'
- 'Talking with you is what I am interested in right now.'

Loss of health – living under threat of death

Two fundamental questions which concern patients facing terminal illness are 'How can I live with this?' and 'How long have I got?'. Coming to terms with living with their condition for an indefinite period and confronting their mortality is a more harrowing process for some than others. Grief may take many forms, including childish and aggressive behaviour. The dietitian who understands the nature of the grieving process is likely to feel less anxious and more able to be empathic. In the following example the dietitian demonstrates this.

> PATIENT: (*angrily*) I suppose you're going to tell me what I've got to eat and what I shouldn't have any more. Well, you'll be wasting your time . . . it's all a waste of time. I don't know how much longer I've got – maybe a few months, maybe a few years. (*his voice breaks, he stops speaking and looks down at his hands which are clasped tightly together. The dietitian maintains her eye contact but does not say anything. She is aware of feeling scared and thinking 'What do I do'? The patient gives a sigh and instinctively she reaches out and puts her hand over his. After a moment he looks up and she notices his eyes are filled with tears*).
> DIETITIAN: (*speaking quietly*) It's all getting too much.
> PATIENT: (*taking a deep breath*) I won't let it get me down. I'm not beaten yet . . . (*and in a stronger voice*) . . . maybe they're wrong about the diagnosis – it's happened before. (*gives her a weak grin*).
> DIETITIAN: (*aware she is mirroring his facial expression and feeling warmth and compassion towards him, removes her hand still maintaining eye contact and not speaking*).
> PATIENT: (*speaking after a few moments silence, in normal voice*) What was it you wanted to tell me?
> DIETITIAN: I came to talk to you about the foods and drinks that will nourish you most. We can do that now or would you prefer another time?

Loss of appetite

Loss of health may lead to a significant loss of weight, as occurs in patients with anorexia nervosa, cancers, acquired immune deficiency syndrome (AIDS), debilitating chronic diseases and post-surgical conditions. In preventing further weight loss the dietitian uses her skills and resources to encourage the patient to eat suitable food and drinks. Her aim is to ensure the patient consumes an adequate energy intake despite a lack of appetite and apathy or antipathy towards eating. When encouragement to eat has no effect the dietitian may resort to persuasion ('Just try to eat a little'), the use of threats ('If you don't eat you'll get even weaker') and giving orders ('You must drink this with each meal'). As she increases her pressure anxiety develops between herself and the patient, creating a barrier in her relationship with the patient (Chapter 6).

When the dietitian's aim (to increase a patient's energy intake) is in opposition to the patient (who has no desire to eat), the dietitian's ability to provide acceptance is tested. If she is unable to accept how the patient is thinking and feeling she cannot demonstrate her understanding (be empathic) and cannot provide the core conditions necessary in a helping relationship. She can extend her ability to provide the core conditions by gaining more understanding of the process her patient is going through. As a result the patient feels more understood and more able to co-operate. Patient and dietitian will then be working together to find a means whereby the patient's needs can best be met, as shown in the following example in which the dietitian focuses on using reflective responding (Chapter 6).

DIETITIAN: I have been thinking about what you told me yesterday – that you don't feel like eating or drinking anything at the moment. Trying to persuade you when you don't feel like it doesn't seem very helpful. I want to help . . . I'm wondering what I can do for you?

PATIENT: (*in flat tone of voice*) Nothing . . . no-one can help.

DIETITIAN: (*gently*) There's nothing anyone can do to help?

PATIENT: (*again in a dull, lifeless tone*) No-one can put the clock back.

DIETITIAN: You'd like to be able to go back to how things were?

PATIENT: (*almost angrily*) Well . . . it'd be a lot better than what's ahead of me. How can I manage now?

DIETITIAN: (*calmly*) You're worried about how you are going to cope.

PATIENT: (*angrily*) Too right I am. I've lost my job, I'm a semi-invalid now – what sort of future is that?

DIETITIAN: (*calmly*) It seems you've lost such a lot and you feel angry about that.

PATIENT: (*in a plaintive tone*) Yes . . . everything's changed.

DIETITIAN: (*calmly*) It seems to you as though everything's changed; (*asks in a questioning tone*) that *nothing* is the same as before?

PATIENT: (*doubtfully*) Well . . . one thing that's not changed – my daughter still visits – she comes whenever she can.

DIETITIAN: (*calmly*) That means a lot to you, doesn't it. We could talk again tomorrow if you would like to?

PATIENT: (*in normal tone*) Yes, I'd like that. You seem to understand and I will try to eat a little this evening.

Not all patients living under a threat of death have a loss of appetite. Patients with human immunodeficiency virus (HIV) infection know only too well that loss of appetite can signal the onset of AIDS and may therefore become obsessive about their eating behaviour. The amount, type and quality of food and drink they consume becomes highly significant to them, for while they are eating and maintaining their weight they are alive and well. The dietitian who recognises the significance that a loss of appetite has for a patient is more able to accept the single-minded attitude with which the patient may pursue their eating behaviour.

Support for the patient and the dietitian

Difficulties occur for both patient and dietitian when either avoid talking about the loss. The dietitian who recognises the signs of grief that the bereaved person is experiencing and understands the process of bereavement is more able to demonstrate the empathy and acceptance that the bereaved person needs. The painful task of grieving often raises conflicts, which may cause someone to seek professional help, and the dietitian may want to consider asking her patient if they have thought of this. Ways and means of referral are discussed in Chapter 4.

Working with patients who are dealing with loss may raise personal difficulties for the dietitian who may herself be dealing with a loss, for example a recent death in her family or loss of health of someone to whom she is close. A patient's experience may trigger unresolved grief for the dietitian, which makes it difficult for her to work effectively with that patient. The dietitian who understands this and appreciates the need to care for herself in order to help others, may consider seeking professional help for herself (Chapter 15). She will want to draw on her network of support and focus on establishing clear boundaries for herself.

Supporting someone who is bereaved is emotionally demanding. Those doing it need to be able to care for themselves and keep their self-esteem high and their level of stress low (Chapter 15). When seeing several bereaved patients the demands on the dietitian are great and she needs to pay careful attention to keeping a balance in her work by having variety in her caseload and her work activities. Support from colleagues is invaluable. The dietitian needs to be able to talk through her concerns about a particular patient with colleagues, and this can add valuable learning for all when it is done with respect for the patient and in a structured way with careful consideration about confidentiality (Chapters 4 and 15).

References

Bowlby, J. (1997) *Attachment and Loss: Attachment*, vol. 1. Pimlico, London.

Bowlby, J. (1998) *Attachment and Loss: Separation, Anxiety and Anger*, vol. 2. Pimlico, London.

Bowlby, J. (1998) *Attachment and Loss: Loss, Sadness and Depression*, vol. 3. Pimlico, London.

Kubler-Ross, E. (2005) *On Grief and Grieving*. Simon & Schuster, London.

Marris, P. (1992) *Loss and Change*. Brunner-Routledge, London.

Worden, W. (2003) *Grief Counselling and Grief Therapy*, 3rd edn. Routledge, London.

Chapter 10

Parents and Children

'A truly great man never puts away the simplicity of a child.'

Chinese proverb

In this chapter I discuss:

- Challenges for the dietitian
- Needs of the child
- The family
- When a child withdraws
- The angry child
- The well-behaved child
- Over-protective parents
- Aggressive parents
- The absent parent
- The dying child

Challenges for the dietitian

Dietitians who work with children face two specific challenges:

- Adapt dietary advice so that it is appropriate for the child concerned.
- Take into account the child's carers (usually parents).

In order to meet these challenges the dietitian needs:

- flexible communication skills so that she can relate to a child of any age;
- awareness of a child's needs;
- familiarity with the ways in which children express themselves.

The degree to which children are dependent on their parents and carers varies with age and development, and increases when a child feels fearful and vulnerable, for example when ill or in hospital. Whether she sees the child alone or with the parent(s), the dietitian who is aware of a child's needs is more able to build a satisfactory relationship with the child.

The dietitian can increase her understanding of the child by being aware of how children fit into their particular family system. For most children this is their family of origin; for some it is the care system in which they live. Each member of the system has their own way of interacting with the others in the system. The dynamics between child and parent(s) as well as the dietitian's own relationship with each, affects the way in which she communicates.

The dietitian can also increase her capacity to understand a child by becoming aware of the way in which a child describes a situation and how he feels, which is likely to be different from that of an adult. The different use of language and way of interpreting situations may mean that empathy is more difficult than with another adult (Burnard 1999).

A dietitian will have a better understanding of how to communicate effectively with children of all ages if she is aware of:

- a child's ability to think and conceptualise;
- a child's need to experiment and learn;
- a child's desire for connection and fear of abandonment;
- a child's striving towards independence.

Needs of the child

A child's physical and psychological needs will vary depending on age and degree of development. Some of these needs are listed in Table 10.1.

Table 10.1   Some needs of a child.

Physical needs	Food, warmth, shelter
	Protection, security
	Physical contact
Psychological needs	Unconditional love, emotional caring
	Acknowledgement, recognition
	Stimulation
	Encouragement
	Acceptance as an individual
	Explanation
	Honesty
	Permission to be sexual

Children need their caretakers to:

- listen to them;
- play with them and have fun;
- provide companionship;
- provide privacy;
- speak on their behalf;
- be reliable;
- provide physical and moral boundaries appropriate to their age;
- allow them time and permission to make mistakes;
- provide structure and routine.

Children in hospital have health workers in *loco parentis*. As a member of the health care team a dietitian needs to be aware of her young patient's needs and her own ability to provide for her patient.

Exercise 10.1

Look at the list of needs in Table 10.1. Which of these needs could you provide for a child aged 10? Imagine yourself providing these, e.g. listening, having fun, being a companion to your patient. How could you demonstrate your reliability and honesty? In what situations do you think you might need to speak on the child's behalf? In teaching a child about diet how do you think you would think, feel and behave when they make mistakes or rebel against the restrictions?

The family

Eating behaviour is inextricably linked with social conditions and relationships within the family, and a child is influenced by the behaviour of parents, siblings, aunts, uncles and grandparents. A change initiated by one member of the family produces a change within the whole family system. The dietitian may find it useful to bear this in mind when advising dietary modification. In the following example Sue, a paediatric dietitian, considers Peter, a 10-year-old boy newly diagnosed with diabetes, within the context of his family.

Sue, Peter and his family

Background
Peter lives with his parents and younger sister. His medical notes indicate that both he and his sister are small for their age and there

is a family history of diabetes. The paternal grandfather developed diabetes in middle age and has since had an amputation of his foot as a result of poorly controlled diabetes. Peter's father has recently been made redundant and his mother works full time as a primary school teacher.

Interview

Sue, the dietitian, sees Peter with his mother. She notes that each time she asks him a question his mother answers on his behalf. Peter does not make eye contact with her and frequently interrupts his mother to contradict what she says. Sue gathers from the conversation that Peter spends a lot of time with his grandfather, a widower who lives nearby. She wonders if it will be helpful to encourage the grandfather's support in managing Peter's diabetes, although she is aware that this could cause friction between mother and grandfather. Sue notices that Peter's father is not mentioned and wonders what kind of a relationship he has with his son and how the stress of the redundancy is affecting the family; also that Peter's mother describes Ann, his sister, as 'fine' and 'no problem'.

Reflections

Afterwards Sue reflects upon the interview. Her first impression is that the family are under a lot of stress; mother seems anxious and controlling, Peter tense and defiant in the face of this, sister possibly feeling a lack of attention, father absorbed in his own problems and grandfather either supportive or demanding. She then thinks about Peter and his mother and jots down the following questions.

Peter:

- How does Peter feel about his diagnosis, about seeing doctors, nurses and herself?
- How will his diabetes affect his relationships with his friends and sister?
- What is his relationship with his father?
- Does Peter feel afraid of him?
- How can she gain Peter's co-operation?
- How much does he know about diabetes?
- How can she tell when he is receptive to information about his diet?
- She thinks that, at 10, Peter should be able to grasp the basic concept of balancing diet, insulin and exercise. Does he know anyone of his own age with diabetes?
- Is he embarrassed at being different from his friends?
- Is he a candidate for a Diabetes UK summer camp at some stage?

His parents:

- How do his parents feel about Peter's diagnosis?
- What knowledge have they already about diabetes and is this accurate?
- How do they think the diagnosis will affect them as a family?
- What role, if any, does Peter's father play in the shopping, preparing and cooking of the family food?
- Would Peter's father come with his wife to discuss Peter's diet?
- What is their relationship with Peter's grandfather?
- Do they see him as a help or a hindrance?

Considerations

Having come up with these questions Sue begins to feel overwhelmed. She wants answers, not more questions! She considers seeing mother and Peter again and instructing them about what he is to eat, what he is to avoid, and how to manage his diet, insulin and exercise. She also considers how to reinforce her instructions by stressing the consequences of not keeping to the diet. Then at least, she tells herself, she will have done her job! She thinks of the others involved in caring for Peter – the medical and nursing staff and his teachers – and notes the following questions:

- Has the dietetic department got any notes on the grandfather?
- Has a colleague in the department given him dietary advice in the past?
- Is it worth getting hold of his medical notes?
- Have the doctors any concerns about both children being small for their age?
- In the case of Peter this may be due to his diabetes, but what about his sister?
- How long has their growth been slowed down?
- Is their size a family characteristic?
- His mother is quite petite but what about his father?
- Is the children's small stature a sign of deprivation or is it of little significance?
- Is anyone else in the team involved with the family?

Making a plan

Sue now feels ready to make a plan of action and jots down the following steps:

- talk to the doctor;
- look up the department records about grandfather;
- see Peter on his own;
- make an appointment to see his mother on her own.

She thinks that more information will help her to decide how best to approach Peter about his diet. She realises that if she can establish a good relationship with Peter it will make it easier for him to learn and will stand him in good stead for his contact with dietitians in the future. She recalls herself at 10 years old when she was in hospital for a tonsillectomy and she remembers how scared she felt in the strange environment and how worried she was about what would happen to her. She remembers counting the hours until she could go home. She wonders if Peter feels anxious like she was.

Next meeting

Sue sees Peter on his own. She focuses on giving him her full attention and actively listening to what he says by using her skills of reflecting instead of questioning which she thinks is likely to seem interrogative to Peter. Her intention is to demonstrate her acceptance and understanding. He slowly opens up to her and begins to talk freely about himself and his family. She learns how much Peter values spending time with his grandfather when he calls in for tea on his way home from school.

Peter suddenly confides in her his fear about having hypos (apparently he had his first the previous day). She focuses on demonstrating her empathy by reflecting 'You feel frightened about having more hypos'. She senses him relax a little and asks him if he feels frightened because he is not sure what to do to prevent one occurring again. He agrees with her. As the time for their interview is drawing to a close, Sue says she will see him at the same time tomorrow and will explain then how he can avoid the risk of hypos by having enough to eat. She asks him if the doctors know about his hypo or if he wants to tell them. He shrugs his shoulders as if he does not care either way. Aware of feeling a little irritated and yet at the same time realising that this may be difficult for him, she says she is willing to tell the doctor on his behalf if he would like her to. He nods his head.

Reflecting upon their meeting Sue thinks she is slowly gaining his trust. She also knows about his fear of hypos and has a lot more information about his eating patterns on which to base her teaching plan (See Exercise 10.2).

Exercise 10.2

Refer again to the list of what a child needs from his caretaker and decide which of Peter's needs were met by the dietitian. If Peter was your patient, how might you meet his needs?

Summary

In the case of Peter, Sue focused on placing Peter in his family context, building a relationship with him and gaining his trust. She gave him time to tell his story and used her skills of active listening to demonstrate her empathy, acceptance and genuineness. Her awareness of being a child helped her be empathic. Her realisation that children's communication is often literal meant that she used words that were unlikely to carry a double meaning. She used the same vocabulary as Peter and made sure that she checked with him that she understood when he used words that had a particular meaning for him and his family. An example of this occurred when he referred to his favourite evening meal as 'plate supper', which turned out to be a specific selection of cold snack foods on his own special plate eaten while lying on the floor in front of the television.

When a child withdraws

In the example above it takes the dietitian some time to establish a relationship in which the child feels safe enough to talk to her. All children can be reticent in this way. This may be temporary or part of a longer period of withdrawal. Whether this be a natural distrust, a sign of depression or an indication of high anxiety, the dietitian does well to note it and inform the medical staff. Meanwhile her difficulty lies in communicating with someone who is behaving in this way. (See Exercise 10.3.)

Exercise 10.3

Imagine yourself with a diabetic teenager who sits opposite you in a slouched position looking down at the floor with a sullen expression on his face. How do you feel? Irritated, uneasy, scared, angry, anxious, nervous? What do you think? Here are some examples:

- 'He's a lost cause'
- 'I don't see why I should bother with him if he can't even be polite'
- 'He may get violent or shout any minute – then what do I do?'
- 'A no-nonsense approach is what he needs – a bit of discipline will make him pull his socks up'

What action would you take?

Guidelines for handling this situation

- Give the child time. Focus on remaining calm and sensing the atmosphere between you. What does the silence tell you?
- Use the silence to focus on creating rapport non-verbally.
- Be aware of how the child is breathing. What does this indicate to you?

It is most likely that the child will break the silence. If he remains silent the dietitian might say one of the following:

- Is there anything you would like to tell me?
- Would you like me to go away?
- If you would rather not talk now I can come back another time.
- You seem a bit scared. Can you tell me about it?

The child who withdraws is most probably feeling anxious, frightened and uncertain and asking himself, 'Can I trust this person?'. The dietitian who realises this can focus on being available for the child (Chapter 5). She then draws on her ability to be empathic and feel respect for the child as a human being who is coping with his current situation in the best way he can. The more genuine she can be as a human being (Chapter 3), the more the child will respond to her and be able to trust her.

The angry child

A child may also withdraw as a way of coping with anger. Silently withholding is one way in which a child can exert his power in the face of authority. Other ways of acting out anger are more easily recognisable, such as shouting, screaming, stamping of feet, throwing toys or food and so on. Dietitians who are unfamiliar with children may feel uncertain about how to deal with anger and rebellion. Those who are parents themselves will be familiar with many ways of dealing with such behaviour. It may not be easy for them to adopt other ways.

Exercise 10.4

Recall a time in your childhood when you felt frustrated and angry. How did you behave? What would you have liked to do to relieve your feeling? How did others behave towards you? Did they ignore you, laugh at you, reprimand you, send you away to another room, punish you by depriving you of something? What do you think would have helped you most at the time? What did you need most?

Guidelines for handling this situation

- Children need their feelings to be taken seriously. Acknowledge that they are feeling angry, thus demonstrating that you accept that they have a right to feel this way.
- Focus on the child's behaviour. Decide for yourself if this is acceptable or not in the circumstances. Let the child know if this is unacceptable to you. For example, 'I see you are angry and I am not willing to listen to you when you swear at me. Feeling angry is OK but behaving in this way is not.'
- Remember that the feelings are valid and real for the child, even though you as an adult may not understand the reason for them.

Young children can be calmed by being held firmly while being allowed to express their anger. This is effective when done lovingly and respectfully, not angrily and punishingly. Physically containing a child provides him with safe boundaries. It is helpful to say to the child, 'You are safe. I am holding you.' Containment is different from the type of physical restraint which serves to compound anger and lead to the child struggling to be free. Although most dietitians are unlikely to find themselves in situations where they need to take such action, they may find it useful to consider.

The well-behaved child

A child who is well behaved can be a delight to work with. However, children may behave in a way which seems 'too good to be true' in an effort to be accepted and liked. The need for approval may be such that the child follows the advice without understanding why it is necessary. Thinking the child has understood her advice, the dietitian may only realise later that this is not the case. Her reaction then is likely to be one of confusion and irritation, thus enabling the child to experience again the disapproval he feared. The child decides he has not been good enough and so increases his efforts to behave well and so the cycle is repeated.

Guidelines for handling this situation

- Focus on how you are feeling. Is your response to this child one of disapproval or irritation? Or maybe you feel anxious to please him?
- Check that the child has understood the information or advice you have given by using open questions (Chapter 7).

- Give the child permission to make mistakes; for example, 'Keeping to a diet is difficult and there will be times when you eat something that is not good for you'.

Over-protective parents

It is natural for a parent to protect their child. There are many examples of situations in which parents perform superhuman feats in order to protect a child. The desire to protect is activated when the parent perceives the child to be in danger. In order to protect their child a parent may behave aggressively or manipulatively towards someone else so as to get what they want for the child. Parents may be demanding on behalf of their child in ways that they would not for themselves.

There are some parents who are overly protective. In their desire to shield their child from what they perceive will be frightening for the child, they think or feel as if they were the child concerned and do not allow the child to express his own thoughts and feelings. When the dietitian asks a child a question in the presence of one or both of his parents, she may find the parents answer for the child instead of giving the child time to answer for himself. She may find herself talking to the parents and ignoring the child. The child may subsequently behave in ways which make it more difficult for the parents to follow the dietary advice. The child who is consulted about the diet is more likely to feel involved and thus be more willing to co-operate. In trying to understand the behaviour and feelings of the over-protective parent the dietitian may find it useful to reflect upon the following questions:

- What are they afraid of?
- How anxious are they?
- What support do they have?
- If their overly protective behaviour is their way of exerting their control over the child, how might they try to control the dietitian?

Guidelines for handling this situation

- Focus on listening and reflecting the parents' concern for the well-being of their child. In this way you will demonstrate your understanding of their need to protect their child.
- Ask them what they want you to do.
- Focus on containing their anxiety by keeping them informed and doing your best to keep to any arrangements that you make with them.

Aggressive parents

Parents may feel aggressive towards children when they are exhausted, when the child is disobedient or ill, or if the parent was a rejected child and has an unconscious impulse to re-enact the experience with their own child (Reinhold 1996). As a result of a parent's aggressive behaviour, a child is likely to feel rejected, hurt and upset and may respond aggressively in turn. On the other hand the child may behave passively and withdraw. Feeling aggressive is part of being human. There are many ways in which we behave aggressively, some of which are overt, others covert. A parent may behave aggressively towards the child or towards the dietitian.

Guidelines for handling this situation

- Maintain eye contact.
- Focus on being calm.
- Consider setting limits.
- Adopt assertive posture – sit or stand upright with arms and legs uncrossed.
- Be brief and to the point when you speak.
- Use 'I' language (Chapters 7 and 14).

The absent parent

A child who is in hospital and whose parents are not there to act as an advocate is likely to feel alone, abandoned, uncared for, anxious, frightened or ashamed. They may cover this by being awkward, belligerent, difficult and unco-operative, or they may be meek, anxious to please, withdrawn, quiet and have difficulty in asking and answering questions.

If one parent is absent, the other who is there with the child may be angry, resentful, and frightened at carrying the responsibility alone. The one who is absent may appear guilty and be anxious to make amends, for example by frequent telephone calls and by sending the child an excessive number of presents. This parent may make excuses for not being there and may rationalise their absence showing great concern and wanting to give the child and the staff gifts or money. On the other hand the absent parent may not make contact at all and may either not know that their child is in hospital or may ignore the situation. The child may feel abandoned by the absent parent and feel a desperate longing for their presence. Such a child may go to great lengths to make contact with the absent parent or may be withdrawn and appear resigned to the situation.

Guidelines for handling this situation

- Be prepared to give time to the child.
- Focus on listening and reflecting feelings.
- Be wary of giving reassurance and making promises, e.g. 'Daddy will soon be here'. You do not know that and it is hurtful to raise hopes that may not be met.
- Be aware that the child may show limited attention to any diet instruction.
- Be prepared for sudden changes in mood.

The dying child

We are likely to feel sadness in response to any death. The death of a person in their eighties is in the natural order of life. The death of a child on the other hand has come about before the expected lifespan has been lived. The circumstances surrounding the death may be distressing, painful and prolonged or the death may be unexpected and sudden. The parents' distress is difficult for all to witness and the dietitian whose child patient has died may be party to the parents' grief. She herself may be more upset than she expected.

The child who knows they are going to die shortly may accept their impending death with a maturity beyond their years. Parents and staff may feel humbled by this and some may be in awe of the child. Being with a child during this time can be a particularly moving, although difficult, experience. The dietitian may be torn between wanting to give the child all it desires in terms of food, and wanting to make sure that any nourishment provided meets the nutritional needs of the body to prolong life.

Guidelines for handling this situation

- Refer to the points on bereavement (Chapter 9).
- Do not assume the child will want to talk to you.
- Respect their right to privacy.
- Watch for signs of tiredness or withdrawal.
- Let the child dictate the pace.
- Find out what the child wants to know first about the issue in question, whether this is about diet or anything else.

- Talk to them normally, not down to them.
- Listen to the child.
- Show respect by not reassuring the child that they will get better when this is untrue. Instead focus on allowing them to express how they feel.

Apart from the first, these guidelines apply to communication with all children. The three below (Burnard 1999) are also worth noting:

- Be aware of pitching questions and responses appropriate to the age of the child.
- Respect the child as a human being who happens to be younger.
- Believe the child.

References

Burnard, P. (1999) *Counselling Skills for Health Professionals*, 3rd edn. Stanley Thornes Publishers Ltd, Cheltenham.

Reinhold, M. (1996) *How to Survive In Spite of Your Parents*, 3rd edn. Mandarin Paperbacks, Northampton.

Chapter 11

Transcultural Communication

'Culture: the acquainting ourselves with the best that has been known and said in the world and thus with the history of the human spirit.'

Matthew Arnold

In this chapter I discuss:

- What is culture?
- Prejudice and its development
- Attitudes and expectations
- Effect of prejudice and cultural differences on communication
- How can we communicate more effectively?
- Talking about food
- Making effective use of an interpreter
- Coping with difficulties

What is culture?

As we grow up we learn values, history, attitudes, practices and beliefs from those around us and from our environment. Those aspects which we share with others form our culture. As children we tend to adopt these cultural factors without question and although we may challenge them in adolescence we think of our own culture as normal. Cultures can be based on many groupings, for example regional, organisational or religious, and are constantly changing and adapting to produce complex variations within a general culture. Our culture becomes such an integral part of our life that we are often unaware of its influence on our thinking, behaviour and attitudes, which can lead to difficulties when we communicate with those from other cultures.

Britain today is a multicultural society. There are occasions when cultural differences seem overwhelming, arousing fear and anxiety. Even so we may make an effort to connect, despite the difficulties. At other times we do not even try. Faced with cultural integration new problems may arise as traditional values and practices are perceived as rejected (Goodinall 1993).

Dietitians are constantly communicating across cultural barriers whether or not they are aware of these. Cultural differences exist not only between dietitian and patient but also between dietitians. Colleagues may have very different cultural backgrounds yet they have had a similar training and are members of the same profession which has a cultural identity of its own. The health service has its own national and local culture, as does a commercial environment, which means dietitians have to adapt to these professional and working cultures while maintaining their own cultural identity, if they are to achieve effective working relationships.

Exercise 11.1

Take a large sheet of plain paper. Draw a circle in the centre to represent your culture of origin and write words or phrases within the circle which describe the cultural norms with which you grew up, such as colour of skin, nationality, country of origin, social class, political allegiance, the television/radio and newspapers you were exposed to, the traditions and customs in your family. Now draw another circle which slightly overlaps this. Write words in this circle to describe the cultural values of your school, e.g. sports loving, academic achievement, emphasis on discipline, strong traditions. Build up other circles in the same way to represent college/university education, work, profession and the different cultures in which you have lived.

As you look at your completed cultural map of interlocking circles, what do you notice? You might want to make notes or talk to a friend/colleague about the adaptations you have made and how the different cultural values have influenced your life.

Developing awareness of our own culture is not easy, particularly when our culture is that of the majority. Those from minority cultures are more likely to have greater cultural awareness. Awareness of how our culture influences us is crucial if we are to be able to 'step outside its constraints and care for others in terms of their own needs' (Schott & Henley 1996).

Prejudice and its development

Prejudice means to prejudge something or someone, that is to form an opinion beforehand. Assigning imagined characteristics and making judgements and assumptions helps us make sense of things around us. The degree to which we do this depends upon our personal experience. We all have prejudices, although we may not like to think this. Depending on our particular culture we may develop prejudices about gender, age, socio-economic group, status, race or sexuality. We think of someone as 'prejudiced' when they are against someone or something, and 'biased' when they are taking another's side or speaking in their favour. Either way we are expressing our prejudice.

Prejudice may not necessarily be racist although racism involves prejudice. There are two kinds of racism – our own personal racism and racism in society as a whole. Racism is 'the conscious or unconscious belief in the superiority of a particular "race", acts of discrimination and unfair treatment whether intentional or unintentional, based upon this belief' (Mares *et al.* 1985). Racial prejudice may be expressed in a 'loud, explicit and often violent manner or in ways which are subtle though no less expressive' (cited in: *Breaking the Silence: Writings by Asian Women* and quoted by Ram Goodinall in his book *Sari 'n' Chips* (1993)).

As adults we may think we would not express such prejudice. However, we may be unaware of how our attitudes towards our own culture and that of another affects our communication. For dietitians living and working in Britain, the dominant culture in the country and in the medical profession frames their view of the world. Anyone not sharing these cultures will be seen as an outsider and perceived as inferior in some way, and this may be difficult for health professionals to acknowledge.

Attitudes and expectations

A dietitian has attitudes and expectations about herself and her patients based on her culture and experience. Patients whose expectations are not met are likely to vote with their feet and not return for future appointments. Relating this to counselling practice, d'Ardenne and Mahtani (1999) point out that when there are great cultural differences between client and counsellor, it is simplest for the counsellor to convince herself that this is due to the client's resistance to counselling. It is much more difficult for the counsellor to consider how her attitudes and expectations might have influenced the client's decision not to return. Clients may sense their counsellor's low expectations of them and so think of themselves as unlikely to succeed. However, they may placate their counsellor by telling the counsellor what they think she wants to hear (d'Ardenne & Mahtani 1999). When there are great cultural differences between patient and dietitian it is simplest for the dietitian to tell herself that the difficulties are due to the patient's resistance to changing their eating patterns, rather than consider how her expectations may have influenced her patient's behaviour.

A dietitian wanting to become more aware of her attitudes and expectations towards a patient may find it valuable to ask herself the following questions (also see Exercise 11.2):

- In what ways am I different from this person?
- In what ways am I similar to this person?
- How do I think this person thinks of me?
- In what ways do I consider myself superior or inferior?
- Am I aware when I feel irritated, impatient and anxious with someone?

Exercise 11.2

Think of a patient you have seen recently whose cultural background is clearly different from your own. Make a note of these differences, e.g. language, gender, age, nationality, race. Recall the scene and how you felt. Were you aware of feeling inferior or superior to the other person? Did this change during the interview? How did you behave when you felt either inferior or superior? What do you think you were afraid of? What do you think irritated you?

Effect of prejudice and cultural differences on communication

Prejudice limits our ability to be empathic, genuine and accepting, that is to provide the core conditions necessary for a therapeutic relationship. It is difficult to empathise with another when we focus on the differences between us. Our acceptance is limited by our desire for the other person to be more like us or a wish that we could be more like them. In other words we judge the differences between us and consider ourselves inferior or superior to the other person.

If we think of someone as inferior to us we tend to behave towards them in a patronising or arrogant way. This may take the form of feeling sorry for them, of seeing them as a victim of their circumstances, or of seeing them as someone to do our bidding and bend to our will. Although they may also see themselves in this way it is not helpful to reinforce these self-beliefs. If we think of someone as superior to us in some way we tend to behave in a subservient manner, anxious to please them and do their bidding. We are likely to put ourselves at their disposal and to set aside our own needs, hoping that in due course they will appreciate our efforts and show their gratitude. When this is not forthcoming we feel resentful, hurt and upset.

When communicating transculturally the dietitian may attempt to break through the barriers by giving her advice in a number of different ways, only to find that her patient seems more confused. The dietitian may go to great lengths to express her sympathy in her desire to be thoughtful and caring, yet she may seem patronising to the patient who then feels angry and resentful. In the following example the dietitian is advising a middle-aged Asian woman who has recently developed diabetes. Although the reader may think the scenario is unlikely, she may recognise some similarities.

> DIETITIAN: (*pointing to the diet sheet*) These are the foods you must now avoid as they contain too much sugar. I know this will be really hard for you especially if you have a sweet tooth. Do you? (*she looks at the patient who drops her eyes and maintains a blank expression*).
> DIETITIAN: (*feeling irritated and unaware of the confusion she may have aroused by her use of the term 'sweet tooth'*) Do you understand what I'm saying? (*The patient keeps silent and continues to look downwards. The dietitian feeling frustrated, now speaks more slowly and raises her voice*) Never mind. The thing is you must not eat sugar any more.

When we think of another person as neither superior nor inferior to ourselves we can more easily accept our similarities and differences in attitude, perception, behaviour and culture. We are more able to offer empathy, genuineness and acceptance, with the result that communication will be more effective and the relationship more satisfying for both dietitian and patient.

How can we communicate more effectively?

A recognition of the values that certain social rituals have for a patient can help the dietitian build rapport. d'Ardenne and Mahtani (1999) explain that the cultural divide may become greater if introductions are not clear, and they point out the significance of names, language, credentials, boundaries and goal setting when working across cultures.

Introductions

When cultural differences are obvious we are likely to feel anxious, irritable and inadequate as we anticipate the difficulties in communication. This is true for both patient and dietitian. Any knowledge about another culture, for example ways of making introductions, helps the dietitian to feel more confident to deal with the situation. In the following example the dietitian is meeting an Asian woman who has recently been diagnosed as having diabetes.

Ann notices the patient's age, traditional style of dress and the fact that she is accompanied by a young man in jeans and T-shirt. From her knowledge of Asian culture she guesses this is the woman's son, that he speaks English fluently but his mother does not, and that her patient may eat a very traditional diet. She is aware that she has a stereotypical situation in mind of the patient leading the traditional role of the older woman in an Asian household and that she is likely to make assumptions because of this.

Talking to someone in an authoritative position is stressful and the dietitian who introduces herself clearly can help a patient feel more at ease. The dietitian who says 'I am Ann Smith' leaves it unclear whether she wants to be called 'Ann' or Ms Smith, Miss Smith or Mrs Smith! Culturally, the patient may feel extremely awkward addressing someone by their first name when they perceive them to be in an authoritative position. The dietitian may also feel uncomfortable when the patient addresses her in a way she had not intended but had inadvertently invited by not making this explicit.

Names are part of our individual and cultural identity and when our names are used correctly we feel accepted. Different cultures have different naming systems and health professionals can cause confusion and offence when they change a style of address to fit in with the British system (Schott & Henley 1996). The dietitian therefore shows respect by enquiring from the patient what they like to be called and, if in doubt, how to spell and pronounce this. Most of us feel irritated when someone consistently mispronounces our name. However, as patients perceive the dietitian to be in a position of power and control, they are unlikely to correct her mispronunciation.

As well as establishing names and any other necessary identity details, it is also useful for the dietitian to explain briefly her role and purpose. This gives valuable information to a patient who may have no idea of the existence or function of dietitians. In doing this the dietitian is establishing her credentials, which may be of great significance to patients whose culture attaches importance to status and position.

Exercise 11.3

Recall the way in which you introduce yourself to patients. How clear do you make it? Do you behave differently with different patients? If there are wide cultural differences between you and the patient, how do you adapt your introduction? How could you experiment with varying the way you introduce yourself and establish your credentials.

Language

Even if a patient is fluent in English their ability to converse will be affected by the stress they feel (Henley 1982). This is true for all of us, whatever tongue we use. We may not be able to articulate what we mean when under stress and our ability to comprehend what is being said is reduced. People often smile a lot, nod as if they have understood, avoid eye contact and remain silent in this situation, or else give brief, inaccurate answers. The dietitian, under stress herself, may mistakenly interpret these signals as signs of comprehension by the patient.

It is important therefore that the dietitian speaks clearly, in concise sentences, uses straightforward language which avoids jargon and colloquialisms and deals with one point at a time. Pictures can be a useful aid. The dietitian needs to check frequently that her patient has understood. Simply asking 'Do you understand?' invites the patient to nod or say 'Yes'. A more effective way is to ask the patient to explain how they would use the information or, if practical, to demonstrate this.

When there is a clear cultural divide it is important to establish the language to be used during the interview. Providing the dietitian has prior knowledge of the patient's country of origin, greeting the patient in their native tongue can be a way of quickly establishing a rapport. 'Welcome, how are you?' may be the extent of the dietitian's language skill. If so it will be necessary to clarify this with the patient and to establish which language is to be used in the conversation. When communicating across a language barrier both dietitian and patient are likely to become weary in a relatively short time. The dietitian who can be flexible allows for this by either covering material in less detail or scheduling more frequent appointments.

The words we use reflect our attitudes and beliefs. The dietitian may have become familiar with using certain words during her clinical work, for example bowels, constipation, urine, and may not realise that these are a source of embarrassment to the patient whose culture does not include their use. Terminology changes over time so that words which were commonly used in the past become superseded by new terms. It is important for the dietitian to be aware of those which are currently acceptable so that she speaks in non-racist language.

Speech patterns and customs

Even though both dietitian and patient may speak the same language, differences in pace, emphasis, intonation, inflexion, volume and conversational style can lead to confusion and misunderstanding in meaning and interpretation. Cultural differences in the use of phrases such as 'please' and 'thank you' may lead to irritation and the conclusion that someone is excessively polite or downright rude. Gaining knowledge of another culture and developing awareness can help a dietitian recognise how and why misunderstandings may come about.

Boundaries

When clear boundaries are established in a relationship both parties are able to relax and communicate more freely (Chapter 4). Some of the practical boundaries may be unfamiliar to someone from another culture. The physical environment, for example where to sit and permission to smoke, are within the control of the dietitian and may impose constraints on a patient whose culture does not share the same social values. The concept of timekeeping may be different for someone from a non-Western culture who may appear for an appointment long after the scheduled time for no apparent reason. Having established the value of clear time boundaries in Chapter 4, the reader may want to reflect upon how she could adapt her approach with someone whose culture does not include these.

Non-verbal communication

Many psychological boundaries in a relationship are established non-verbally, for example in the way we position ourselves in relation to the other person, and in our gestures, eye contact and facial expression (Chapter 5). There are cultural differences in non-verbal communication (Morris 2002) and the dietitian needs to ask herself if a patient's non-verbal signals are specific to their culture before she assigns a particular meaning to the communication.

Goal setting

As with time keeping, goal setting may be an unfamiliar concept to someone from another culture (d'Ardenne & Mahtani 1999). The idea of achieving a target weight, for example, may be a concept the patient is unwilling to adopt. Although it may be the dietitian's objective the patient may have in mind something else, for example to obtain the dietitian's help in dealing with a social problem. The dietitian's skill in clarifying expectations is essential if a mutual purpose is to be established (Chapters 2 and 4).

Talking about food

As dietitians know only too well, food has a significance for most people far greater than its nutritional value. Different cultures have different customs associated with food, which may be based on moral values and health or social, religious and spiritual needs. Customs around food preparation, cooking and eating are many and varied. However strange a custom may seem to the dietitian it is important that she remembers that it is familiar to the patient for whom that custom is part of their cultural identity. To talk about changes in diet is particularly stressful for someone whose cultural practices are very different from the majority culture. When giving dietary advice to a patient of another culture a dietitian needs to be particularly aware of the significance that any change she suggests may have for the patient. She can do this by:

- using her skills of active listening (Chapter 5);
- clarifying, by reflective responding, what are the patient's customs and practices (Chapter 6);
- being aware when she is assuming these for a patient because of her knowledge of the patient's culture. Although background knowledge is useful information it is not necessarily true for a particular individual. To assume that it is can increase the likelihood of being perceived as patronising.

Making effective use of an interpreter

An obvious difficulty of transcultural communication occurs when we do not speak the same language. Interpreters are likely to be unofficial, for example relatives. This gives rise to difficulties concerning suitability, confidentiality and accuracy of translation. Bias and distortion can be introduced by the interpreter as well as exploitation of the patient (Shackman 1985). Many dietitians will be familiar with the situation of a middle-aged female patient who does not speak

English and who has her young son with her to act as interpreter. Not only is there the age difference but also gender and status differences. The culture gap in this case is enormous, making any meaningful communication unlikely.

When a relative is not present to act as an unofficial interpreter, it is often the practice to ask a stranger of the same nationality, for example a nurse who is working in the outpatient department. It is tempting to assume that because two people originate from the same continent they speak the same language and dialect. It is important to check that this is the case before beginning the interview. In India, for example, there are many different languages and even more dialects.

Interviews using interpreters take longer. Extra time is needed beforehand to:

- discuss with the interpreter what the interview is about;
- explain how the interview will be conducted;
- encourage the interpreter to interrupt and check if they are in any doubt about what is being said.

Being in the position of interpreting for someone is stressful. Unofficial interpreters may feel coerced into doing it and may be resentful. A clinic nurse may feel she cannot refuse to act as interpreter because it is expected of her, yet it is not recognised officially as part of her duties. On the other hand she may feel responsible for and protective of the patient. When communicating through an unofficial interpreter, the task becomes easier if the dietitian uses words that are unambiguous and speaks in sentences that are clearly structured.

In her book *The Right to be Understood* Jane Shackman (1985) draws on her experience of using interpreters in her work with refugees and highlights the importance of checking the following points:

- Does the interpreter speak English and the client's language fluently?
- Is the interpreter acceptable to the client (the same sex, similar age)?
- Is your client prevented from telling you things because of his/her relationship with the interpreter?
- Are you creating as good a relationship as possible with your client?
- Is the interpreter translating exactly what you and your client are saying or are they putting forward their own views and ideas?
- Does the interpreter understand the purpose of the interview and what her role is within it?
- Does the interpreter feel free to interrupt you to ask for clarification or point out problems?
- Are you using simple, jargon-free English?

- Is the interpreter ashamed or embarrassed by the client?
- Are you asking too much of the interpreter?
- Are you allowing the interpreter enough time?
- Are you maintaining as good a relationship with the interpreter as you can?

Coping with difficulties

There is much to think about when working transculturally. Dietitians can work towards more effective transcultural communication by gaining knowledge of other cultures and developing awareness of how their own society and culture have influenced them. Appreciation of both the differences and the similarities enables a move towards greater acceptance of one another. When communication becomes difficult it is tempting to blame the other person and their culture, or to blame ourselves for being inadequate. Blame leads to guilt, frustration and helplessness in the face of the cultural divide. The dietitian who recognises when she is blaming herself or her patient is more able to focus instead on finding some point of greater understanding, thus building a bridge between her and her patient.

Ways of building bridges

(1)   By becoming more aware:

- Note the thoughts and feelings you experience when you see a person from another culture or racial background.
- Reflect on the meaning that these thoughts and feelings have for you.
- Consider the culture of the person before naming their behaviour as normal or abnormal.
- Exercise your imagination by thinking of yourself in the place of the other person, leading their life as you understand it.
- Think about your own cultural background – how would you describe yourself to someone from another culture?

(2)   By recognising:

- when a particular non-verbal behaviour represents a cultural difference rather than an individual variation;
- the fears that your patients bring with them that increase their prejudice;
- the differences between you and another where these exist.

(3) By focusing on:

- establishing rapport (Chapter 5);
- understanding your own racial and cultural prejudices and the way they influence your communication;
- involving the patient's family and community networks appropriately;
- using their language and knowing when and how to use an interpreter.

References

d'Ardenne, P. & Mahtani, A. (1999) *Transcultural Counselling in Action*, 2nd edn. Sage Publications, London.

Goodinall, R. (1993) *Sari 'n' Chips*. South Asia Concern, Sutton.

Henley, A. (1982) *Asian Patients in Hospital and at Home*. Oxford University Press, Oxford.

Mares, P., Henley, A. & Baxter, C. (1985) *Healthcare in Multiracial Britain*. National Extension College, Cambridge.

Morris, D. (2002) *Peoplewatching – A Guide to Body Language*. Vintage, London.

Schott, J. & Henley, A. (1996) *Culture, Religion and Childbearing in a Multiracial Society – A Handbook for Health Professionals*. Butterworth Heinemann, Oxford.

Shackman, J. (1985) *The Right to be Understood: A Handbook on Working with, Employing and Training Community Interpreters*. J. Shackman, available via email: janeshackman@waitrose.com.

Chapter 12

Working with Difficulties in Physical and Mental Health

'What man is he of wit so base
that wears both his eyes in a case
for feare of hurting them it is
and I doe find it not amisse'

From: *A Booke of Merrie Riddles* (1631)

In this chapter I discuss:

- Minority needs as part of society
- The effect on patient and dietitian
- Resources for the dietitian to develop
- Physical difficulties
  ○ Hearing
  ○ Sight
  ○ Speech

  ○ Mobility and movement
  ○ Appearance
  ○ Invisible disabilities
- Mental health
  ○ Recognising anxiety and depression
  ○ Thinking about eating distress
  ○ Hearing suicidal thoughts – how can I bear it?

Minority needs as part of society

Those who, through accident, illness, age or circumstances of birth, have a loss of ability to function physically or mentally, have certain special needs which differentiate them from those who are able to function fully. Such differences may carry a stigma even in an apparently tolerant and liberal-minded society. There is increased awareness in recent years of issues associated with various mental and physical problems, and a variety of articles in magazines and pro-grammes on television and radio which aim to raise consciousness and disseminate information. Self-help groups have exerted pressure to increase public awareness and some policies have been implemented and statutory requirements made for the provision of necessary facilities. However, there is a long way to go before those needs which are particular to a minority are accepted as an integral part of society.

Loss of ability to function affects both mind and body, including verbal and performance skills. Problems with mental health can affect someone physically, and someone with physical disabilities can be affected emotionally and mentally. Misuse of alcohol, drugs and food may develop as a way of coping and these strategies in turn can become disabling behaviour for some. Many people also live with some degree of chronic pain. This in itself is disabling and can affect all areas of a person's life. As a result a person may become more withdrawn or increasingly aggressive. Relationships are likely to become strained and tense and may break down altogether resulting in increased isolation.

Physical problems can affect hearing, sight, speech, mobility, movement and appearance. There are disabilities which people have had from birth, for example spina bifida, and those which develop slowly as a result of progressive disease, such as multiple sclerosis. There are also those which are the result of sudden trauma, for example a road traffic accident. Learning difficulties caused by illness or infection since birth or during the perinatal period are experienced by those with Down's syndrome, cerebral palsy, dyslexia and epilepsy. People with learning difficulties are not necessarily ill. They require the same everyday services as anyone else in order to live in the community. They also have specific requirements to assist them with living in the community, as may those with physical disabilities, and like others they may suffer from problems with mental health.

Exercise 12.1

Note on a piece of paper the people you know, either in a personal or professional capacity, whom you consider to have a physical or learning difficulty or a problem with mental health. Make notes on the nature of the difficulty, how you think this affected them, any special needs they have, and any remarks you have heard made about people with this difficulty.

The effect on patient and dietitian

Reactions to loss of ability may be so intense that some people become unable to function socially, professionally or personally. Some may feel anger, fear and resentment, sadness and despair, hopelessness and powerlessness, and anxiety and depression. Others may deny feeling any such emotions. Physical difficulties may compound the effect of the original problem; for example, a patient who has suffered a stroke may become incontinent, which can lead to embarrassment and a fear of social contact and being away from home. Isolation and depression can lead to ever-increasing withdrawal, and lack of activity and exercise may develop. Antidepressants may be prescribed, some of which can have physical side-effects.

People learn to cope with their difficulties in many different ways. Some coping skills lead to a degree of adjustment and acceptance which makes life manageable. Other means of coping, such as misuse of alcohol or food, increase problems in the long term and compound the difficulties.

All areas of human life can be affected in some way as a result of physical and mental health problems, including eating behaviour. Dietitians who are concerned with giving dietary advice to patients and carers will be well aware that the problem of maintaining a healthy weight is greater when opportunities for physical activity are limited. Patients may have gastro-intestinal difficulties and may have special needs associated with managing any practical problems connected with food preparation and eating.

The dietitian's attitude and previous experience and her own individual emotional response will affect the way in which she communicates with a patient, whatever their difficulty. There will be times when many dietitians may doubt their ability to help the patient. As well as a sense of inadequacy some may also feel frustrated and helpless when ideas and suggestions do not seem to be accepted and acted upon by the patient.

As with cultural differences (Chapter 11), physical and learning difficulties are likely to trigger prejudice (Exercise 12.2). This has been succinctly defined as 'an attitude that predisposes a person to think, feel, perceive and act in favourable or unfavourable ways towards a group or its individual members' (Secord & Blackman 1974). In becoming more aware of how our own attitude predisposes us to behave towards those with physical and mental health problems, we become more able to offer the core conditions for a helping relationship (Chapter 3). The extent to which the dietitian can provide the core conditions for a particular patient depends on her ability to acknowledge, accept and respect the similarities and differences between herself and another.

Exercise 12.2

Read the following statements one at a time. As you do so be aware of any thoughts and feelings which arise. Can you 'own' this feeling, that is accept it as your own and not attribute it to anyone or anything else. You may like to do this exercise with a partner so that you can take it in turns to talk about your response while your partner listens.

Statements:
- People in a wheelchair shouldn't let themselves get so fat. They've no self-discipline.
- Someone who can't masticate properly won't miss a lot because they can have most food liquidised.
- As he's blind he won't be able to eat fish because of the bones – we don't want him to swallow any.

You may want to add other statements as these occur to you.

Resources for the dietitian to develop

Internal resources

Working with patients who are depressed and who have little energy is demanding for the dietitian and it is important that she take active steps to maintain her own sense of well-being (Chapters 14 and 15). When working with people whose needs are different from her own, the dietitian has many opportunities to use her imagination. Creativity and improvisation are resources to draw upon when helping patients overcome a problem. Extending herself imaginatively and becoming aware of any feelings of fear, anxiety, sadness and frustration helps a dietitian build on her ability to be empathic. The following questions are useful to reflect on:

- What is it that this person most needs from me now?
- What listening skills shall I focus on?
- What message (if any) do I want to put across?
- How can I say this openly and directly?

Exercise 12.3

Here is the outline of a situation in which a dietitian has been asked to help. First, read it through then list as many difficulties as you can think of which may arise in this situation for the patient, the daughter and the dietitian. How might you manage if you were the patient, the daughter or the dietitian. What would you want as the patient, the daughter and the dietitian if someone were to offer you help.

An elderly widow has recently had a stroke which has left her partially paralysed down one side, including her face. She is unsteady on her feet and it was not considered safe for her to live on her own. She moved in with her daughter, since when she has gained a considerable amount of weight. She has developed arthritic pains in her knees. Her daughter has a part-time job, a husband and two teenage children.

External resources

Self-help groups provide valuable support for those with many different mental and physical problems, and their families. Information, advice and opportunities to reduce isolation through telephone helplines, local groups and newsletters are available for many. These and other organisations can be a useful resource for dietitians to pass on to patients and relatives (Appendix 2). Some provide training for health professionals and carers.

Other professional carers such as occupational therapists, physiotherapists, social workers and members of the community mental health team can also be a valuable resource for dietitians. Primary health care teams are increasingly using the services of a counsellor for help with emotional and interpersonal difficulties. A dietitian may find there are local counselling services and groups which offer valuable support. Some patients may appreciate information about these.

Physical difficulties

This section highlights areas which are of concern when communicating with those who have difficulty with hearing, sight, speech and mobility. The degree to which any disability affects a person's daily life is very individual and may not be apparent to others. Altered physical appearance, such as disfigurement or the presence of a prosthesis, has an effect on the dietitian and the patient, and the way in which they cope with this affects any interaction between them.

Hearing

The patient may be hard of hearing in one ear only. If the dietitian establishes that this is the case she can take steps to ease any difficulty by making sure she is sitting on the patient's hearing side. The patient may wear a hearing aid, in which case the dietitian may not have to raise her voice. The dietitian can make it easier for a patient to lip-read if she makes sure she is looking at them when speaking and does not cover her mouth with her hand.

Exercise 12.4

Recall a time when you were with someone with a hearing difficulty. How severe was their disability? How did it affect you? How did they cope with it? How did you cope with it?

The dietitian helps by:

- sitting on the hearing side of the patient;
- turning to be face to face;
- making eye contact;
- writing her message if necessary;
- either being able to use sign language herself or knowing someone who can.

Sight

People who are blind or partially sighted learn to focus on other senses such as sound and touch. Surroundings which are familiar are easier to manage. Change evokes anxiety and this may be more acute for a blind person than for a sighted one if the change involves dealing with unfamiliar surroundings. Sighted people do not have to raise their voices when talking to someone who cannot see. Although to do so seems ludicrous it is often what happens. A blind person knows when someone is talking and looking away from them because they are so attuned to alterations in voice.

It is helpful therefore to maintain eye contact as if the blind person were sighted. The dietitian may not find this easy as people who are blind from birth may use many head movements when speaking or listening. This can be disconcerting for the sighted person if they are unaware that this is normal behaviour for the other person.

It is helpful if the dietitian makes a point of describing any actions she is taking to the blind person so that they know what is happening.

For example, the dietitian who explains to her patient that she is about to make some notes is keeping the patient informed about what she is doing. The patient can then understand the reason for the break in conversation.

The dietitian helps by:

- being aware of the volume of her voice and adjusting this if too loud;
- being prepared for unusual facial expressions and head movements;
- looking at the patient even though she knows the patient cannot see her;
- saying what she is doing so that the patient knows what is happening;
- offering her arm rather than grabbing that of the patient when guiding them;
- considering making a tape recording of her dietary advice to give to the patient instead of a leaflet or diet sheet;
- being aware of the significance of familiar and unfamiliar surroundings and routines for the patient when proposing any changes in lifestyle and alterations in eating patterns.

Exercise 12.5

Recall a time when you were with someone whose sight was impaired. How severe was their disability? How did it affect you? How did they cope with it? How did you cope with it?

Speech

People who stammer or who have difficulty in co-ordinating thought and words need time in which to speak. The listener may feel embarrassed, impatient, irritated and possibly afraid that they too may begin to stammer. They may also feel anxious to help and respond by completing the sentence on the speaker's behalf. When this happens some people may feel annoyed that they have not had an opportunity to express their own thoughts and feelings. Other people may feel they have been helped and supported in their struggle to express themselves.

Those who stammer know they do so and if the dietitian is able to convey in some way that she can accept this they are likely to feel valued as an individual. The dietitian demonstrates her empathy and acceptance by employing her skills of active listening. Paraphrasing and summarising help to clarify what has been said for patient and dietitian. As a result the patient is likely to feel more relaxed and may be able to speak more fluently.

The dietitian helps by:

- allowing enough time for the interview and keeping calm;
- being aware that she may be perceived as impatient and patronising when she completes words or sentences for her patient;
- asking the patient what they would like her to do when they stammer – complete the word for them or give them time to speak.

Exercise 12.6

Recall a time when you were with someone with a speech impediment. How severe was their disability? How did it affect you? How did they cope with it? How did you cope with it?

Mobility and movement

Holding cutlery and kitchen utensils can be a painful problem for someone with arthritis, a fractured wrist or arm or any physical disability affecting their hands and arms. Disabilities that affect mobility and movement make shopping, food preparation, cooking and eating more difficult. The time and energy needed to do tasks that previously may have taken a fraction of the time and effort give rise to frustration and fatigue. This is as true for other parts of the body which are affected by disability as for arms and hands. Those suffering from chronic back pain, for example, know only too well the disabling effect of this and the effort involved in continuing to perform daily activities.

Most people learn to feed themselves at an early stage in childhood. Losing the ability to do this strikes deeply as we are once more dependent for our survival on those who care for us. Developing the self-confidence to use gadgetry is a valuable step towards gaining a measure of independence, which in turn builds self-confidence. A patient who is confident enough to ask for help when it is needed and who has able-bodied and willing friends, family and neighbours is likely to manage more effectively than someone who withdraws from social interaction.

The dietitian helps by considering the following questions when interviewing patients with difficulties with mobility:

- Does the patient need a wheelchair?
- Is the chair a suitable height?
- Do they need an arm for support?
- Is their a clear passageway for them or are there obstacles which if moved would make it easier?

Exercise 12.7

Consider the room in which you usually see patients. Reflect on how user-friendly this is for people with difficulties in mobility and movement. How easy is the access? Are the chairs adequate for their needs? Is the room so small and cluttered with furniture that they might have difficulty negotiating their way around?

Appearance

Facial and other disfigurements, whether due to congenital malformation, burns, skin disease or stroke, are disabling. Learning to live with disfiguring disabilities is difficult for both the person affected and their friends and family. The dietitian who meets a patient with severe burns, for example, may feel shocked by what she sees, even though she may have been told to expect this. The patient may find their self-confidence severely undermined by what has happened to their appearance and this can lead to an increasing dependence on others. As with other disabilities, social interaction, recreation and work opportunities are likely to be affected.

Exercise 12.8

Recall a time when you met someone who was disfigured. How severe was this? How did it affect you? How did they cope with it? How did you cope with it?

The dietitian helps by:

- letting the patient know she wants to hear about their needs;
- focusing on seeing beyond the other's appearance;
- talking about their disability with them if they raise the topic;
- getting support for herself in coping with her own emotions.

Invisible disabilities

Disabilities such as facial disfigurement, amputations, blindness and so on are more or less obvious to another person. There are also disabilities which are hidden from view, for example ileostomies, colostomies and permanent sites for injection of intravenous drugs. The dietitian may not know of the existence of these unless she is told by the patient or reads this information in the medical notes. She is likely to have more difficulty in imagining the effect of a disability on someone's life when the disability is not apparent to her.

Mental health

Difficulties with mental health can happen at any age and result in much distress, not only to the individual sufferer but also to family and friends. The majority of people with mental health problems are living in the community. Care is based on needs being met by community services, and hospital treatment for acute illness when someone is unable to cope with and understand society.

Depression and *anxiety* are the two areas of mental health which dietitians are most likely to encounter. Although 10% of the UK adult population report significant depressive symptoms every week only 1% admit to suicidal thinking (Davies, Naik & Lee 2001). Although the number of actual suicides is low there are many other self-harming behaviours which are widely practised by sufferers to cope with their intense distress. Substance misuse, such as drug taking, alcohol misuse and compulsive eating, is perceived by sufferers as a way of dealing with their problems. Many health practitioners on the other hand perceive this behaviour as the problem itself. A dietitian who appreciates this difference in perception will realise that, when she invites patients to change their eating behaviour, she is asking them to give up a behaviour that (for them) has been a solution. Giving this up can seem an extremely risky course of action to the patient. Feelings may surface and be so intense and overwhelming that the patient harbours suicidal thoughts. When these are expressed to the dietitian she needs to know how to respond.

Recognising anxiety and depression

Most people recognise anxiety and associate their experience of this with certain stressful events in their lives. Some people live with a continual degree of anxiety and have difficulty in recalling a time when they felt relaxed. Anxiety affects the way in which we relate to and communicate with others. Becoming more aware of the signs of stress within ourselves and others alerts us to the need to relax (Chapter 15). The dietitian can help an anxious patient to unwind by employing her skills of active listening (Chapters 5 and 6). Patients who are extremely anxious may demand more in terms of time and attention than the dietitian feels able to give. It is important for the dietitian in this situation to set clear boundaries (Chapters 4 and 8) and follow these through.

Many people at some time or another will have described themselves as depressed. This may be a normal response to a life event, for example feeling depressed following a bereavement. When prolonged and intense, depression gives rise to loss of energy, lack of concentration and lack of interest, and mood changes beyond those normally experienced. People may find their sleep patterns disturbed and their appetite altered. They may discover that daily activities take a long time and require more effort than they can sustain. Their digestive system may be affected giving rise to symptoms such as heartburn, indigestion and constipation. They may suffer headaches and other non-specific aches and pains. As well as feeling ill, those who have suffered depression know what it is like to despair, feel hopeless, helpless and frightened and to consider suicide. Psychologist Dorothy Rowe, who has written extensively on the subject of depression, describes it as 'the most terrible sense of being trapped and alone in some horror filled prison' (Rowe 1996).

In the face of another's problems it is easy and tempting to give suggestions and solutions which would appear to resolve the problem. The dietitian may respond in one of the ways mentioned below in the belief that she is acting in the patient's best interest. Such responses, however, do carry a risk of creating a barrier between the dietitian and her patient. For example:

- Reassurance, e.g. 'Don't worry. You'll soon get your appetite back.'
- Remonstrating, e.g. 'Come on now – pull yourself together.'
- Persuading, e.g. 'All you need to do is eat just a little more.'

People who are depressed find the idea of any action difficult and demanding. The dietitian who responds with reassurance, remonstration or persuasion is failing to recognise this. The dietitian who can demonstrate her understanding through her skills of active listening and reflective responding is likely to be perceived as empathic. When a dietitian is able to show acceptance in this way she is providing emotional support. In the following example the dietitian is seeing an elderly patient with arthritis and diabetes who was widowed the previous year.

DIETITIAN: How can I help?
DIETITIAN: (*after a long pause in which she observes the patient sitting very still, looking down at the floor and not making eye contact with her*) It's not easy to know how to begin, is it?
PATIENT: (*after a pause sighs deeply*) It's all so difficult. I just don't know what to do for the best.

DIETITIAN: You have some ideas but are not sure which one would work best?

PATIENT: I go round in circles. It's all too much effort.

DIETITIAN: You're finding it all too much.

PATIENT: (*begins to cry quietly*) I don't know how I can carry on.

DIETITIAN: You don't know how to carry on. (*pause in which she notices the patient nods silently*) Would it help if we talked about your ideas and worked something out together?

PATIENT: (*wipes her yes and looks up for the first time*) Maybe . . . maybe it would help . . . I managed all right to start with but just lately . . . everything seems pointless . . . why should I bother to eat when I don't feel hungry?

DIETITIAN: You managed at first and now there doesn't seem any point in trying.

PATIENT: No point at all . . . I'm not hungry and now Jane doesn't come in.

DIETITIAN: You used to eat with Jane?

PATIENT: No. Jane . . . my neighbour always came in . . . regular as clock-work she was . . . to check I was all right and to see if I wanted anything.

DIETITIAN: And now Jane doesn't come any more.

PATIENT: No. She's moved away – gone to live with her sister.

DIETITIAN: You miss her visits.

PATIENT: Yes. I can't get out much you see . . . if only I could (*sighs wistfully*).

DIETITIAN: You'd like to get out more if that were possible?

PATIENT: Yes, but how?

DIETITIAN: How can you eat out more? Maybe we can come up with some ideas together?

PATIENT: I had heard about a lunch club in the town for people like me . . . (*the dietitian writes this idea down and together they come up with several ideas*).

DIETITIAN: Now we've got some ideas the time has come to choose one to try out. Which would be your first choice?

PATIENT: I like the first one best. Do you know anything about it?

DIETITIAN: I have a list of lunch clubs in my office. Would you like me to send you a copy so you can contact one?

PATIENT: Yes please – I feel better now having talked to you.

There are many different paths this conversation could have taken. The important feature is that the dietitian provides support, which the patient values. By using her skills of reflective responding the dietitian creates a relationship in which the patient feels she can trust the dietitian sufficiently to talk to her. Through her approach the dietitian demonstrates her respect and acceptance of the patient and her willingness to give support without providing solutions. Instead the dietitian uses skilful questioning to help the patient think of ways around the problem. By inviting the patient to articulate thoughts and feelings she gives the patient an opportunity to clarify what help she needs from others.

A patient may describe themselves as depressed or the dietitian may suspect they are feeling this way. How can she tell if this is more than the everyday 'down' feelings that are common to being human? Patients who report a major change in mood, say they have been feeling depressed for some time or give an indication that life is no longer worth living or that nothing seems to make any difference or matter any more, are giving signals to alert the health professional (Kennedy 1981).

Faced with a situation in which communication is difficult, the dietitian may think to herself, 'I can't get through to this person'. Feeling stuck in this way is frustrating and enervating and it is tempting to ask more and more questions in an effort to get the patient to talk. The dietitian who notices a 'flatness' about someone who has not responded to encouragement or other invitations to talk and who is alert to the signals already mentioned, needs to draw this to the attention of the patient's family doctor, consultant or a clinical psychologist. Dietitians who are working in the community are able to liaise with the community mental health team. See Chapter 4 for issues surrounding confidentiality and referral.

Thinking about eating distress

Despite much research there seems to be no straightforward answer why some people use food in an abusive way which may even be life-threatening, and no definitive way of addressing the distress which results (Buckroyd 2005). Extensive interviews with patients reveal that most believe their problems arise in childhood and are associated with some form of trauma (Goodspeed Grant & Boersma 2005). Culture too plays a part. The culture of consumerism, the focus on body image, the widespread availability of food and possibly the addictive potential of excessive intakes of fats and carbohydrates, are likely factors (Buckroyd 2005). Whatever the cause, the effect is intense emotional distress for the patient. Eating food, initially a source of comfort and a way to manage distressing feelings, then becomes more and more difficult to control. Fear of losing control grows so that the idea of giving up a strategy that had previously worked and is familiar, even though known to be potentially life-threatening, is daunting to say the least. Thus the excessive consumption of food which may have started as a way to ease emotional pain and manage feelings, becomes the source of additional emotional distress.

Helping someone to break an established pattern of disordered eating behaviour is demanding work. Someone who binge-eats, for example, may find themselves increasingly unable to cope socially, psychologically and physically. Their relationship with food becomes a focus which can affect their relationship with others as well as influencing their behaviour in social and work situations. They may take excessive doses of laxatives or resort to self-induced vomiting to control their weight. In this way they can successfully maintain an outward appearance of normal weight. Breaking an established pattern of disordered eating behaviour is therefore demanding work for both patient and dietitian.

Dietitians who can appreciate in some way the ambivalence felt by their patients will approach their work with them with greater sensitivity. The focus of treatment for eating disorders has changed from a blanket prescription of willpower, dieting and antidepressants to include behavioural modification. Behavioural programmes produce initial weight loss but this is not sustained (Wilson & Brownell 2002). Cognitive-behavioural therapy programmes are being developed to help patients adhere to diet and exercise (Cooper, Fairburn & Hawker 2003). As understanding of the deep emotional distress underlying the misuse of food has developed, there is greater interest in counselling and therapy. So where do dietitians fit in? When making a nutritional assessment the underlying social and psychological issues may become apparent. The dietitian who has an understanding of the wider background in which people currently struggle to find a meaningful role in life, will realise something of the issues of self-image and self-nourishment which are a fundamental concern of those in eating distress (Waskett 1993).

In assessing whether or not a patient is ready or willing to change their eating behaviour, the dietitian will find it helpful to apply the stages of change (Prochaska & DiClemente 1986) described in Chapter 4 as a framework. She will also find it helpful to carefully consider what she is asking her patient to do as explained above. When thinking about how to help her patient the dietitian using a counselling approach will focus first on stage 1 of Egan's model of the helping process (Egan 2004) (Chapter 4) that is, on building the relationship with the patient, paying particular attention to clarifying boundaries. The quality of the helping relationship she can build with her patient and her competence in managing their working arrangements so that the patient feels secure enough throughout, will determine to a large extent the outcome of their work together.

Whether anorexic, bulimic or eating compulsively the patient needs to feel accepted. She will probably have difficulty in talking about her behaviour and feelings as her need for secrecy and sense of shame, guilt and anger may be so great. She is likely to feel ambivalent about her ability and desire to change her eating behaviour. The dietitian who recognises her patient's needs and can offer help in a way which meets these is providing in-depth support (Table 12.1).

Table 12.1   Meeting a patient's needs.

What a person needs	What the dietitian can offer
A need to talk	A listening ear
To feel safe	Clarity about time and confidentiality
To test if they can trust	Genuineness, acceptance, patience
To be recognised	Acknowledgement
To feel in control	Choice, e.g. of appointments, of changes the patient could make
To be accepted	To take her patient seriously and go at the patient's pace

It is important that the dietitian respects her patient's difficulty and does not push her into talking about what she does with food and how she feels. The dietitian who remains aware of the deep pain of her patient, even when this is not apparent on the surface, will be more able to convey her respect. Her ability to do this may be challenged at times as her patient tests the dietitian's commitment to help, for example by missing appointments or arriving late or unexpectedly. At times the dietitian will probably feel frustrated, inadequate, impatient and angry with her patient. Remaining clear about what is happening while showing acceptance, gentleness and patience, is demanding. The reader is recommended to read again Chapters 3 and 4, to use the review in Chapter 8 (Table 8.2) to help her monitor what is happening in her relationship with her patient, to concentrate on using her skills of active listening and reflective responding as described in Chapters 5 and 6, respectively.

At some stage the dietitian may realise that her patient needs more time and skilled help than she can provide and may consider offering alternative support, for example referral to the local eating disorders team. Dietitians who are members of teams providing an eating disorders service may learn some ways of working interactively with patients by observing clinical psychologists and psychiatrists. Dietitians may feel uncertain about the boundary between dietetic advice and psychological intervention. Using counselling skills responsibly involves assessing and monitoring one's ability, skills and competence and recognising when one is working beyond one's limits (Chapters 4 and 15). A dietitian can learn to do this by having adequate training in counselling skills and skilled supervision as an integral part of her work.

Hearing suicidal thoughts – how can I bear it?

Whereas in the past dietitians were most unlikely to hear a patient talk of harming themselves, nowadays it seems likely that, at some time in her career, a dietitian will hear her patient expressing thoughts of harming themselves in some way. Understandably most helpers feel initially shocked, anxious and helpless when a patient expresses such thoughts. Suddenly we imagine ourselves as less competent and find ourselves thinking: Are they serious? What do I do? What do I say? The following information, based on training material developed by the Counsellors and Psychotherapists in Primary Care (Hudson-Allez 2004), and reproduced with permission, is included to help dietitians at such a time.

Steps to take:

- Take any indication of suicide (or other forms of self-harming) seriously – you may be tempted to ignore it, pretend you didn't hear it or make a light-hearted comment.
- Help the patient to talk – this will enable you to find out more and make a risk assessment.
- Discuss with the patient how they could get help.
- Give the patient a phone number to use in an emergency, e.g. Samaritans.
- Tell the patient that you are required to inform their doctor – it is best if you can agree together what you will say or write.
- Discuss the impact that this has had on you with your supervisor/ mentor/manager.

Useful information to pass on

An example is given in Chapter 4 (p. 41) in which the dietitian clearly states the limits of the confidentiality she can offer. In this example she states that she will hear what her patient has to say in confidence unless she considers this puts her patient's health at risk in which case she needs to inform her patient's doctor. Patients expressing suicidal thoughts are clearly putting their own health at risk. The dietitian who then refers to any agreement about confidentiality that she has previously made with her patient, will be demonstrating that she is taking her patient's remarks seriously. The dietitian then needs to encourage the patient to talk. This gives her an opportunity to find out the following about the patient:

- How long he has been having suicidal thoughts.
- Whether he has ever acted upon these thoughts.
- Whether he has ever planned how he would take action.

- Whether he can think about the effect his action may have on others.
- Whether he regularly practises other forms of self-harm, e.g. misuse of alcohol, drugs or food.
- Whether he is taking medication on which he could overdose, e.g. antidepressants.

Encouraging patients to talk may seem like encouraging them to think more actively about suicide and that this will increase the likelihood of an attempt. However, a patient will continue to think about self-harm whether or not he talks about it. When he does talk and if he experiences being accepted, believed and to some extent understood, he may feel less alone, at least for a while.

Health professionals have a duty of care to patients to pass on information that would enable others to provide appropriate care. With this in mind the dietitian will need to convey to the patient her responsibility to inform the patient's doctor so that an assessment of risk can be made. Table 12.2 lists some indicators of risk.

Table 12.2   Indicators of risk.

A history of self-harming	Previous suicide attempts
Expressing suicidal ideas	Considering/planning action
Expressing high levels of distress	A family history of suicide
Recent significant life events	Major physical injury/disability

Use of these indicators of risk can help the dietitian frame the information she gives the doctor. For example she could write:

'During my interview with Mr. Jones he became very distressed when talking of recent life events and told me he has been having suicidal thoughts for the last month. Although he says he would not act upon these thoughts I am concerned that he discusses the issues with you.'

Exercise 12.9

Imagine you are interviewing a patient who expresses suicidal thoughts. Note how you feel and what you are thinking. What would you say in response? What would you write in your notes? Who would you turn to for support?

Responding to a patient who talks of suicide is further explored in the section 'Middles' in Chapter 13.

References

Buckroyd, J. (2005) Editorial. *Counselling and Psychotherapy Research.* 5, 187–190.

Cooper, Z., Fairburn, C.G. & Hawker, D.M. (2003) *Cognitive Behavioural Treatment of Obesity: A Clinician's Guide.* The Guilford Press, New York.

Davies, S., Naik P.C. & Lee A.S. (2001) Depression, suicide, and the national service framework. *British Medical Journal.* 323, 808–809.

Egan, G. (2004) *The Skilled Helper – A Problem Management Approach to Helping,* 7th edn. Thomson Wadsworth, Belmont, CA.

Goodspeed Grant, P. & Boersma, H. (2005) Making sense of being fat: a hermeneutic analysis of adults' explanations for obesity. *Counselling and Psychotherapy Research.* 5, 187–190.

Hudson-Allez, G. (2004) *Suicide – Hearing It and Bearing It. A Training Day Developed by Counsellors and Psychotherapists in Primary Care.* Bognor Regis, West Sussex.

Kennedy, E. (1981) *Crisis Counselling – The Essential Guide for Non Professional Counsellors.* Gill & MacMillan Ltd, Oxford.

Prochaska, J.O. & DiClemente, C.C. (1986) Towards a comprehensive model of change. In: *Treating Addictive Behaviours: Processes of Change* (eds W.R. Miller & N. Heather). Plenum, New York.

Rowe, D. (1996) *Breaking the Bonds – Understanding Depression and Finding Freedom.* Harper Collins, London.

Secord, P.F. & Blackman, C.W. (1974) *Social Psychology,* 2nd edn. McGraw Hill, New York.

Waskett, C. (1993) *Guidebook for Counsellors – Counselling People in Eating Distress.* British Association for Counselling, Rugby.

Wilson, G.T. & Brownell, K.D. (2002) Behavioural treatment for obesity. In: *Eating Disorders and Obesity* (eds C.G. Fairburn & K.D. Brownell). The Guilford Press, New York.

Chapter 13

Putting It into Practice

'Practice makes for true knowledge'

Chinese proverb

In this chapter I describe:

- Interview 1 – beginnings
- Interview 2 – middles
- Interview 3 – endings

In this chapter, extracts of three different interviews between dietitians and patients are used to illustrate how the interview framework can be applied in dietetic practice. Counselling skills are applied in each interview. The exercises at the end of each interview are designed to help the reader reflect upon, comment on and learn from each example.

Interview 1 – 'Beginnings'

Asha is a recently qualified dietitian working in a district hospital. Today she is in the diabetic outpatient clinic. The time allocated for the appointment is 20 minutes. The patient she is about to see is Alan, aged 45, who was diagnosed five years ago. His blood sugar levels are controlled by diet alone. He has been referred to the diabetic clinic because these levels have been erratic for the past six months.

Asha is preparing to meet Alan. She reads his medical notes which give his medical and social history, details of the medication he has been prescribed and the results of blood tests and other examinations. She has been asked to assess his diet and advise as she considers appropriate. As she has not met Alan before and knows little about him, she lets her mind wander for a moment imagining him as overweight, a smoker, a drinker, a workaholic who sees little of his wife and children. She mentally shakes herself aware that the real person may not be like this at all. She glances around the room. It is small, windowless and contains two identical upright chairs, a clock on the wall and a computer on the desk along with her files, notepad and pen. It is a functional, characterless room, but it is quiet and not too stuffy and has easy access to the main outpatient waiting area. She thinks it could be more welcoming, but she has known worse. She moves the chairs so they are at an angle and a comfortable distance apart thinking that she will indicate to Alan to sit in the one furthest from the door and she will have the other which will give her a corner of the desk to lean on when taking notes. She glances at her watch, and realising she is on schedule, takes a few moments to focus on being calm and relaxed. She walks into the main waiting area and looks around. Several people, both men and women are waiting. Which is Alan? She notes three likely people and approaching them says in a clear voice 'I'm looking for Alan Bull.'

'That's me.' A man gets up and moves towards her. She smiles in acknowledgement.

'Please come this way', she says and leads the way towards the interview room. Motioning him to one of the chairs she says, 'Please take a seat.' She sits down, and looking at him feels surprised. Alan is not at all like she had imagined. She sees a man of average height and build, short dark hair greying at the temples, who is clean shaven, and is wearing a grey jacket and blue open-necked shirt. She thinks he has a pleasant face although he is frowning a little at the moment and sitting almost on the edge of the chair.

Asha wonders if he is feeling anxious and decides to concentrate on putting him and herself at ease. Smiling, she says in what she trusts is a welcoming manner: 'Hallo. I'm Asha, one of the dietitians here. We've not met before and I'm wondering if you've talked to a dietitian before about your diet?'

'Yes. Some time ago though. Just after I was told I had diabetes I think it was.'

Asha wonders if there is a record of this in the department. She wants to assess what he knows about diet as a means of controlling his diabetes and says, 'I'm wondering what you remember of that meeting – what you found helpful? Or maybe it wasn't helpful at all?' She decides to pose both possibilities trusting this will help him acknowledge honestly how he found the previous interview.

'I don't remember much about it except being given a lot of information about how my sugar levels would go down if I didn't eat sweet things. So I don't – I've not got a sweet tooth anyway so it's no great problem.'

Asha feels a little rebuffed by the somewhat abrupt tone in which he makes this last remark. Realising they are at Stage 1 of the helping process and her task is to build a helping relationship, she decides to apply her skills of reflective responding.

'So you haven't found it difficult to avoid having sugar and foods containing a lot of sugar.' She then decides to risk asking a direct question to encourage him to identify what he perceives is the problem. She says, 'What do you think has been the biggest difficulty?'

'Well I guess it's when I feel sort of dizzy. It's not every day but when it happens people tell me to have something sweet and then I feel better. It's odd really because that's the very thing I'm meant not to have', Alan replies frowning slightly.

Needing to clarify what he has said Asha summarises saying 'You've found the most difficult thing to cope with is the feeling like dizziness that happens sometimes and you've discovered you feel better when you eat something sweet but you're thinking that doesn't make sense because sweet foods are what you've been told not to have.'

'Absolutely. Can you explain it?'

Asha recognises this as Alan's way of challenging her. It is also an opportunity to take a diet history and move into the next stage of the interview. However, she remembers she has not clarified the time they have available nor how they are going to spend it. Neither has she explained her agenda which is to assess his diet and advise him appropriately. She thinks his dizzy spells may be signs of hypoglycaemia and realises she can explain how he can avoid these by managing his diet. To do this she will need to assess his diet and advise him accordingly thus fulfilling her own agenda. She recognises too that she needs to continue to build a helping relationship and that they are likely to need another appointment to complete their work. Glancing at the clock she says 'I'm aware we have 15 minutes left today. How would it be with you if we spend some of that time sorting out how your dizzy spells seem to respond to taking sugar – something you know it is best if you don't eat – and leave time for you to ask me any questions you want to about your diet? We also need to discuss whether you would like another appointment and if so when we can arrange that'.

'Sounds good to me', he says with a small smile, sitting back in his chair.

This concludes the beginning section of the interview. Exercise 13.1 allows the reader to reflect on this stage of the interview.

Exercise 13.1

The interview framework
In the extract above what tasks appropriate to the beginning stage of the interview does Asha focus on? Are there any tasks that you consider appropriate to this stage which she has left out? How could Asha have handled these differently? What are your reasons for these suggestions?

Communication skills
- What assumptions, if any, does Asha make and how do they help or hinder the progress of the interview?
- What significance, if any, do you attach to Asha's non-verbal communications? Identify the different types of response Asha makes during the interview, e.g. summarising. How might you have responded differently and why?
- How does Asha build a helping relationship? How successful do you think she is?

Many dietitians find it helpful to role play situations such as the interview between Asha and Alan with a colleague. In doing this it is valuable to enact both roles so that you get an experience of being both the dietitian and the patient. Allow time to discuss with your colleague and to debrief before switching roles and at the end of the exercise.

Interview 2 – 'Middles'

Kate is a senior-grade dietitian working in the community. She is meeting Jenny, aged 33, for the first time. Jenny, who has a body mass index (BMI) of 38 kg/m², has been having episodes of binge-eating. The time allocated for the interview is 45 minutes. Below is a summary of the first 15 minutes.

Summary of the beginning stage

Kate's first impression was that Jenny was anxious and her somewhat dishevelled appearance led Kate to wonder if she did not care much about the impression she made. Maybe she simply had too many demands made of her? She appeared slightly overweight and spoke quickly as though she should hurry although Kate had already clarified how long they had together and Jenny had nodded in agreement. Kate had concentrated on putting Jenny at her ease and had explained to her that she had been asked to assess Jenny's diet. When asked why she had sought help with her eating Jenny had explained that she had been struggling to control her weight for the past two years since the birth of her second child. In Kate's opinion Jenny needed to lose 3–4 kg, however, Jenny had declared she should lose twice that. She had returned to hairdressing 18 months ago and enjoyed the company of colleagues and clients. Although a large proportion of her earnings went on child care this had become less recently as her eldest child was now at school. She had gone on to say she was 'sick to death' with not being able to get back to the weight she had been before she had her children and badly wanted Kate to help her do this. They had agreed they would spend most of their time today assessing how best to help Jenny. Kate had felt alarmed when Jenny had used phrases like 'sick to death' and she had explained to Jenny that whatever she said was confidential between them but that if she considered Jenny's health to be at risk she would want Jenny's agreement that she could talk to her doctor about these concerns. Jenny had said this was all right with her.

The middle stage

The interview now continues. Kate invites Jenny to tell her more about her eating patterns and Jenny starts to tell Kate about a meal she had the previous weekend with friends from work to celebrate a birthday. Her voice is low, she speaks quickly with her gaze fixed on the wall between them.

'I'd been really looking forward to going out – I hardly ever have the chance these days. All day I'd been telling myself I would only have a main course and a coffee but I knew I'd blown it when everyone started ordering desserts. I ordered the chocolate fudge cake – I really love it – how could I resist? Anyway a while afterwards I began to feel stuffed to bursting point – sort of bloated and I knew I shouldn't have eaten it all. Then before we all left the restaurant I went to the loo and caught sight of myself in the mirror. I looked awful! I felt awful! I wanted to die I felt so bad. One of my friends came to get me – I'd been there so long – and we then went home. I'm not sure how I got there but the next thing I remember was waking up and vowing to myself I wouldn't eat another thing ever again. So you see the whole evening was a disaster. I reckon I'm a pretty hopeless case!', Jenny gives a hollow laugh.

Kate notices the tears in Jenny's eyes and is aware of feeling increasingly anxious herself as she listens. Is Jenny saying she wants to commit suicide? Kate wonders how much, if any, alcohol Jenny drank that evening, whether she has had similar experiences in the past and whether she had made herself vomit or taken laxatives while alone in the toilet at the restaurant. How should she respond to Jenny? Kate focuses on being calm and keeping her eyes on Jenny's face she speaks slowly, her voice at normal volume and her tone gentle.

'I can see you feel very upset and I hear you say you think the whole evening was a disaster. You seem very ashamed of eating a dessert – so ashamed you even wished you didn't exist anymore.' She pauses noticing Jenny is looking down at the floor. When Jenny doesn't say anything Kate continues, 'I'm thinking it took a lot of courage for you to tell me what happened.' Jenny looks up with a surprised expression. 'Courage? I've never thought of myself as having courage. It's more that I'm desperate.' She sighs. After a few moments she continues, 'I can talk to you – you don't tell me what I should and shouldn't do all the time like some people.'

Kate registers this remark as an indication that Jenny is building trust in her relationship with Kate. She notes also Jenny's acknowledgement that she is feeling desperate. Is this an indication of her motivation to change or another indication of suicidal thoughts in which case Kate will need to refer her for an assessment of her mental health. She needs to know more and so says to Jenny, 'I'm glad you feel you can confide in me and I want to help you. When you say that after the meal last weekend you felt desperate and you wished you could die I'm wondering whether this is the first time you've felt so bad or whether you often think about suicide? Can you tell me more?'

'Yes, quite often. I wouldn't actually do anything though 'cos of the children. My doctor thinks it's because I'm depressed and I suppose he's right. I feel worse about myself when I can't control my eating. I guess that's why he sent me to see you.'

'So your doctor knows you've been having suicidal thoughts which seem to be more frequent when you don't seem to be able to control what you are eating.' Kate wants to clarify what Jenny perceives as her goal. 'You want to be able to control what you eat?' Jenny nods. 'Is this a problem for you all the time or only on particular occasions like last weekend when you eat out with others?'

'Oh I guess it's pretty much in my mind a lot of the time.'

Jenny continues to tell Kate how low she has felt since her second child was born two years ago, how tired she is all the time, how isolated she feels and how worried she is that she is not being a good mother. The more Kate hears of Jenny's life the more she realises that Jenny's difficulties are compounded by her circumstances. She also realises they have ten minutes left. She decides to focus on making a contract with Jenny. She starts by summarising their interview so far.

'Jenny I'm aware we have ten minutes left today and I'd like first to recap on what we've talked about. From what you tell me you have been finding life a struggle for a long time, anxious that you are not managing well enough and feeling alone with your problems. You try to control yourself by restricting what you eat 'cos while you can do this you feel better about yourself. The problem is that when you then eat something you've told yourself you shouldn't, you feel so bad about yourself that you eat even more and so end up feeling even worse.' Kate pauses and sees Jenny nod. She continues, 'I'm wondering how best to help you. We could arrange another meeting to talk more about how you could adjust what you eat to lose a little weight on a balanced diet. Maybe I could help you think how you could say no, for example to the dessert in the restaurant, so that another time you have some new ways of coping if you think that would help?' Jenny nods and Kate continues, 'I think we will need three, maybe four meetings to do this – how would that be with you?'

For the first time Kate sees a smile flit across Jenny's face. She says to Kate, 'I'd like that.'

Kate wonders if Jenny would be willing to consider other sources of help for her depression, isolation and low self-worth. She continues 'I'm also wondering what you think about talking to someone, for example your health visitor or a counsellor about how you feel so depressed?'

Jenny frowns slightly. 'Do you really think that would help? Sometimes I think I'm going mad – I think I do need help but who do I go to?'

Hearing Jenny pose this question, Kate decides to take the opportunity to explain to Jenny that her family doctor would be the best person to ask. Most medical practices nowadays have access to the services of a counsellor albeit only for short-term counselling.

The extract ends here as they move into the ending stage of their interview which is spent sorting out future appointments, giving Jenny an opportunity to say how she has found the interview and to ask Kate any questions. The reader is invited to read through the text again, and complete Exercises 13.2 and 13.3 which focus on the interview framework and using the person-centred approach, respectively.

Exercise 13.2

(1) Using the summary of the beginning stage of the interview name the tasks that Kate has completed.
(2) What tasks has Kate fulfilled in this middle stage of the interview?
(3) If you were in Kate's place how would you conduct these tasks?

Exercise 13.3

(1) How does Kate demonstrate each of the core conditions of empathy, acceptance and genuineness?
(2) What effect does this have on her relationship with Jenny?
(3) How aware is Kate of her own feelings? How does she use this awareness?

In Exercise 13.4 the reader is invited to consider how Kate could apply her knowledge of cognitive-behavioural therapy (CBT) (Chapter 7) at their subsequent meetings.

Exercise 13.4

Refer to the section 'Helping someone towards clearer thinking' in Chapter 7. Read again the interview between Kate and Jenny and then complete the following.

(1) Note the words that Jenny says which indicate distorted thinking.
(2) Take each example of distorted thinking in turn and consider what assumption Jenny could be making which underlies this thought, e.g. 'I hardly ever have the chance.' Possible assumption: 'I'm a failure.'
(3) Suppose you were to make similar assumptions and think as Jenny does. What replacement thoughts would you develop?

It is helpful to discuss ideas and role play with colleagues possible ways in which you might help Jenny towards clearer thinking.

Kate reflects on her interview with Jenny

After the interview Kate feels concerned about Jenny, and she is unsure of how she handled the interview and how to proceed next time. She decides to use the framework for review outlined in Chapter 8 (see Table 8.2). Aware of confidentiality Kate accepts that any notes she makes are for her own personal use and that she will destroy these once she finishes the exercise. She thinks 'What do I know of Jenny?', and notes on a blank piece of paper: Female, 33 years. What is Jenny's health like? Kate writes 'Binges, slightly overweight since first pregnancy, expressed suicidal thoughts in our interview and said she often feels like this. Said her GP [general practitioner] knows about her suicidal ideation'.

Kate now begins to feel more enthusiastic about doing this review and moves on to the section on social information. She notes 'Hairdresser

– enjoys job and company'. Looking at the next points she suddenly realises Jenny said nothing about a partner or husband or the father (or fathers) of her children or other members of her family, her home or anyone who provides support. Although she mentioned the friends she went out with for the meal Kate is struck by this gap in her knowledge of Jenny. For a moment she berates herself thinking she should have asked Jenny but then she thinks to herself 'It's interesting in itself that Jenny did not mention any of this'. She notes on her paper 'Talked of friends but no mention made of partner/family. What about support?'. Under presenting issues Kate notes that Jenny had come to see her because she was 'desperate' to control her eating and considered her problem to be her inability to get back to her pre-pregnancy weight. Kate, however, wonders whether Jenny's problem lies in her depression and that food has become significant for her as a way of coping with whatever it is that is making her feel depressed.

Kate now turns her attention to the section of her review on working together. First what did Jenny want from her? Kate recalls Jenny saying 'I want to get back to the weight I was before I became pregnant' and this being twice the weight loss Kate thought necessary. Kate wonders if Jenny was underweight before becoming pregnant, maybe having a history of a disordered relationship with food. So was Jenny wanting Kate to help her explore this? Kate begins to feel anxious and out of her depth. She asks herself 'What can I offer Jenny?', and feels pleased that she was able to be clear with Jenny about the number of appointments they could have and how they could use them to help Jenny feel more in control. Jenny had seemed pleased about this. Kate also thought she had helped Jenny by raising the idea of her getting help with her mental state and felt pleased that Jenny had said she would think about this. On the whole Kate considered their relationship so far had developed satisfactorily. She notes on her paper 'history of issues with food and weight preceding pregnancies. Has agreed to four appointments to explore ways of making food choices including diet assessment. Will think about counselling for depression'. As she reads through the notes she has made, Kate feels pleased she has done this exercise. She finishes off by thinking about the points she wants to consider further as her work with Jenny progresses: continuing to build a helping relationship and possibly drawing on her knowledge of CBT to help Jenny think differently about her reactions to food and her weight. She thinks Jenny could benefit from more support than the few sessions she is offering, especially concerning the non-diet related issues, and she wants to help Jenny access some counselling through her GP if that is what Jenny decides she wants.

Interview 3 – 'Endings'

Ann is a senior dietitian with a particular interest in group work and weight management. Savita, aged 48, has been a member of Ann's weight management group and a month ago completed a course of ten sessions during which her BMI dropped from 55.3 kg/m^2 to 50.5 kg/m^2. This extract is from an individual 30-minute follow-up session which Ann routinely offers to each person in the group.

Ann welcomes Savita.

'How are you', she enquires.

'Not too bad,' says Savita. 'It seems strange coming here without the others.'

'Yes doesn't it,' agrees Ann. 'As we discussed at our last group meeting I see today as an opportunity for us to complete the work we have done together and to say goodbye. I'm wondering how you feel about this being our last meeting?'

'A bit anxious to tell you the truth' says Savita. 'How am I going to manage on my own? I'm doing OK at the moment but what if I can't keep it up – there's a big family wedding in three months time which could be a difficult time for me. I don't want to slip back to old ways of eating.'

'Hmm . . . a difficult time – not only the wedding itself but all the preparations too . . . you're feeling anxious when you think about it. And now the group has finished I imagine you're thinking you're going to be more on your own?' Savita nods and Ann continues, 'Would it help if we discussed this more in a few minutes?' Savita nods again and Ann continues, 'I think it would be helpful first if we take a broad view and look back to when we first met, how you were then . . . over the work you have done on yourself since and the changes you have made to your eating habits . . . I'm wondering how you see yourself now?'

Savita takes a deep breath giving herself time to think. She speaks slowly and thoughtfully. 'Well when I first came to see you I felt very bad about myself – I hated the way I looked but I couldn't see how I could do anything about it – I felt really stuck. Now I can see ways I can do things differently – like I don't have to always eat whatever I can lay my hands on whenever I feel fed up. I can talk more about how I feel instead of stuffing it down inside myself.' Savita smiles at Ann, who realising the significance of what Savita has said, wants to affirm this for her. She says, 'So making the connection between feeling miserable and eating has been important for you and you are now finding another way to deal with your feelings.' Savita nods and Ann continues 'I wonder what helped you realise this?'

Savita replies without any hesitation, 'Oh it was hearing some of the others in the group – going to those meetings was really useful once I'd plucked up the courage to join.'

Ann is surprised as she remembers Savita being one of the quiet ones in the group. Savita continues 'I learned so much from the others – as they talked I thought I'm not the only one – other people feel like me and do dreadful things with food too. I began to feel less ashamed.'

'So feeling better about yourself has helped you take more care of yourself – to change the way you were using food?', Ann wonders if she has understood correctly.

'Yes I guess so. It's a struggle though. Some days are easier than others but I try to take one day at a time.' Savita looks at Ann who nods encouragingly. She continues quickly. 'It's hardest when I'm too much alone or when I get very tired or days when everything seems to go wrong. Then I worry I haven't lost more weight and I think I should have and the doctor will be cross and I will have failed. There I've said it . . . I feel so . . . so . . . inadequate.'

Ann feels moved. Savita is sharing her vulnerability with Ann who says gently, 'The times when the struggle seems hardest is when you feel isolated and miserable and nothing seems to go right? That's when you feel bad about yourself? And then want to eat?' Ann feels as though she is struggling herself at this point. She watches Savita nod miserably. 'And how is it different on another day?'

Savita smiles a little. 'When I am doing something I want to. Like the computer course I've just started – it's only once a week but it's good. And someone has asked me to help them with catering for a party they are having – I feel so pleased to be asked. They said they wanted traditional Indian dishes and I do enjoy cooking – especially for others. And when I'm busy and enjoying myself, eating isn't something I want to do – I forget about it! Hard to believe but it's true!' They both smile sharing Savita's moment of pleasure.

'You said how much you learned from being in the group – what, if anything, do you think you have learned about food and health that is useful to you?', Ann asks.

'Oh the discussions we had about healthy food – what was healthy about it and new things to try. Actually it was good to hear that many pulses, fruits and vegetables – the foods I have always used – are healthy and that others want to try them – that made me feel good! I do know though that too much ghee and sugar is not good. I liked the class when we each brought a favourite dish – several people said how much they liked mine!'

'It sounds as though being part of the group where you felt appreciated and valued and you could learn from others was a rewarding experience for you and has given you confidence. And now that support has finished what do you think will take its place?', Ann asks.

'Yes it's difficult – but the best thing is I do keep in touch with two people from the group. We help each other – we talk on the phone. It's good to have someone I can call if I want to talk and I feel pleased too when they call me – it's like we're in it together.'

'So being able to talk to others who you know will understand is important – and you will have this support at the time of the wedding?' Savita nods thoughtfully.

'Yes that's true – I do think I'm going to find the wedding itself and the time leading up to it stressful. It's going to be a challenge but I can see now that I can get through it with the support of my friends. I do hope so – I've come this far I'm determined to keep going this time. Thank you for all your help – it's meant a lot to me.'

'Thank you. I wish you well. I think you will be able to draw on all you have learned to help you – keeping in touch with the others is important too for them and for you. I am referring you back to your doctor now letting him know we have completed our work together. What would you like me to say?'

'Oh . . . hmm . . . well I suppose that I have lost weight and that it has all been very helpful . . . and I hope to keep it up – something like that.'

'How about I say Savita has completed the weight management course which she found helpful and supportive. She succeeded in losing weight – her BMI has changed from 55 to 50 and she is determined to continue with her healthy eating plan.'

'Yes that's fine. Ann – thank you so much for your help.' Savita gets up preparing to leave and smiling warmly at Ann holds out her hand. Ann shakes her hand. 'Goodbye Savita – I have truly enjoyed our work together. Good luck with all your plans.' She shows Savita to the door and closes it behind her.

Exercise 13.5 is designed to help the reader review the ending stage of the interview and apply the review of the dietetic interview (see Chapter 8, Table 8.2).

Exercise 13.5

Using the questions in the review of the dietetic interview (Table 8.2) at the end of Chapter 8 and the extract from the interview here imagine yourself in Ann's place. Make notes reviewing Ann's last interview with Savita.

You may find it helpful to review Ann's work with a colleague using your notes, also to explore what you have learned from doing the exercise that you could apply in your own interview procedure.

Points to make

As explained in Chapter 12 and raised in the second interview in this chapter (Kate and Jenny) dietitians may feel uncertain about the boundary between dietetic counselling and psychological intervention. Review and assessment of her ability, skills and competence are essential if the dietitian is to be able to recognise when she is working beyond her limits (Chapters 4 and 15). In Part 4 the themes of support and ongoing personal and professional development are further examined.

Part 4

Areas for Personal Development

Using counselling skills requires the dietitian to consciously focus on another person while at the same time being aware of what she is thinking, doing and feeling. In becoming more aware and open to herself she becomes more open and aware to others. The further along this path she goes the more effective she becomes in applying her skills. She needs support in this journey of personal development which is an integral part of being able to work interactively with others. The process of personal development is an ongoing one which demands time, energy and commitment, and at times is painful, arduous and challenging, but it can also be joyful and satisfying, bringing immeasurable rewards and significant personal learning (Rogers 2004).

Although it is intended that the dietitian uses the material in Part 4 for her support and personal development, she may also take from it ideas which she considers appropriate to use with patients. Some find books about personal development are informative and supportive and a selection are included in Appendix 1. Some find much to learn from personal development courses and workshops that are becoming increasingly available. However, there is no substitute for experience and dietitians are recommended to use as many opportunities as they can to apply the skills and ideas outlined in Part 4. Many people find that keeping a journal or reflective diary is a useful tool. This may take the form of the reflective diary that dietitians include as part of their portfolio or it may be a separate and more intimate account of personal thoughts and feelings.

In Chapter 14, I explore ways in which the dietitian, faced with some difficult situations in her work, can further her ability to communicate effectively by developing assertiveness skills and strategies for dealing with difficult situations. Such personal development includes building self-esteem, enhancing self-awareness and managing personal stress.

These subjects, together with giving support to others and receiving it for oneself, are explored in Chapter 15.

Reference

Rogers, C. (2004) *On Becoming a Person*. Constable & Robinson, London.

Chapter 14

Dealing with Difficult Situations at Work

'An event has happened upon which it is difficult to speak and impossible to be silent.'

Edmund Burke (1789)

In this chapter I discuss:

- When the dietitian is confronted
- Developing assertiveness
- Steps towards becoming more assertive
- Giving criticism and praise
- Receiving criticism and praise
- Dealing with aggressive behaviour
- An ABC for handling confrontations

Difficult situations arise from time to time between dietitian and patient and between dietitian and colleague who may be another dietitian, another health professional or a member of staff in a subordinate or superior position. Misunderstandings and miscommunications often lie at the heart of any difficult situation. Our willingness to continually examine and develop our communication skills enables us to learn something from each experience. Examples of difficult situations faced by dietitians are given as illustrations throughout this chapter.

When the dietitian is confronted

When we feel threatened or attacked it is difficult not to react defensively and respond either passively or aggressively. Remarks and comments which are perceived as criticisms reinforce self-doubt and result in a lowering of self-esteem (Chapter 15). Frequently such confrontations are expressed manipulatively and the dietitian may not be sure exactly what is being challenged. Sometimes the dietitian is challenged by the patient. For example, a patient may complain about the diet and yet could be upset about the system in the clinic/ward, the dietetic/medical profession as a whole, or the health service in general. The dietitian may somehow feel personally criticised. When a patient says accusingly, 'It's up to you to make sure I get the right food' the dietitian's first reaction is likely to be one of anxiety. At other times remarks are made by colleagues, managers and health professionals from other disciplines. The suddenness of an attack can be a shock and the dietitian may be so taken aback that she responds in a seemingly calm manner. Once the initial shock has worn off she may respond passively or aggressively.

After an incident in which a patient has sworn, shouted or made an abusive remark at the dietitian she will most likely feel especially anxious. She may or may not want to talk about this to others and may rationalise her feelings by telling herself that it is not important, the patient did not mean it, it could have happened to anyone. She may blame the patient or herself for provoking the outburst and may feel afraid of a similar occurrence in the future. She may think that it is over and done with, yet continue to experience disturbing dreams. Debriefing after such an event is necessary so that the dietitian may use the experience constructively. It is of great value for the dietitian to have colleagues with whom she can talk and who can offer her support. Guidelines are given in this chapter for dealing with verbal abuse and risky situations. Chapter 15 gives further guidelines for giving and receiving support. Exercise 14.1 is designed to help the reader become aware of when she has been in situations of this sort.

Exercise 14.1

Think of occasions when you have felt confronted, challenged or criticised. You do not have to limit yourself to interactions with patients. There are likely to be times with ward staff, medical staff and colleagues. How did you respond? How did you feel? What did you do?

'You don't understand'

Fortunately, it is not every day that dietitians are confronted with verbal abuse. Confrontation is more often indirect; for example, the comment 'You don't know what it's like' may be made or implied as when a patient says, 'I've been a diabetic for 40 years and I know what I can and can't have – my life has got to be tolerable after all!'. The dietitian who is aware of the hidden message contained in such remarks and is able to confront this openly and directly is less likely to feel manipulated.

Obvious differences in age, gender or culture may encourage a patient to believe that the dietitian cannot understand their situation. The dietitian is often considerably younger than the patient. Or she may be a great deal older, for example a middle-aged dietitian and a teenage girl with anorexia. A recently qualified dietitian in her twenties inevitably will have less experience than someone who has been qualified and practising for a number of years.

The dietitian will also have a different life experience from her patients. So the remark 'You don't know what it's like' is accurate. No-one can know what it is like to be another person and in their particular situation. Any experience we have had may be similar but cannot be the same. However, although we may be a different age, gender, social class and culture, we have all experienced anger, fear, sadness and joy. The extent to which we can empathise with another's feelings in any particular situation is the extent to which we can demonstrate our understanding.

The most effective way to demonstrate understanding is by reflective responding (Chapter 6). When demonstrating empathy in this manner we provide one of the core conditions for a therapeutic relationship, as described in Chapter 3. The following response is one way in which the dietitian could demonstrate this:

> PATIENT: I've been a diabetic for 40 years and I know what I can and can't have – my life has got to be tolerable after all!
> DIETITIAN: You have managed your diabetes for many years and know what you like and don't like to have. (*tentatively*) You seem worried that any changes I suggest means your diet will become more restricted?
> PATIENT: (*nods*) Yes – that's just what I was thinking!
> DIETITIAN: (*stating her purpose*) That's not my intention at all. I want to help you to eat as much variety as possible while at the same time having a healthy diet.

Difficult situations with colleagues

When faced with a difficult situation three questions are worth considering carefully (Dickson 2004):

- What is happening?
- How do I feel about it?
- What would I like to be different?

The following are three examples of dietitians considering different difficult situations.

Nicky, a basic-grade dietitian working in a district hospital, has learned that an inpatient has not been receiving the food supplements she has arranged for him to have. He had seemed so ill and grateful for her interest in him. She had gone to a lot of trouble to ensure he would be given the supplements. She feels annoyed to learn he had not been getting these. She also feels afraid that she might be at fault although she cannot understand how this could be. She is sure she followed the correct procedure. What shall she say to him? What shall she say to the nursing staff or the doctor? She wants to appear professional and confident and to be able to sort out the situation satisfactorily so that it does not happen again. However, she is anxious that she will be nervous, and appear weak and ineffectual.

Tina, a community dietitian, is thinking about a situation with a general practitioner (GP). It has come to her attention that he is handing out very-low-calorie diet sheets to patients, which she considers inappropriate. She feels annoyed when she realises patients are getting conflicting advice. She feels anxious about speaking to him because he has been short-tempered with her in the past. She is also worried that somehow he will turn the tables and she will end up thinking of herself in the wrong. When she speaks to him this time she would like to be able to express her concerns clearly and calmly, to feel at ease with him and to gain his co-operation.

Jo, another community dietitian, is meeting Fran, a practice nurse. A diabetic patient had said to Jo that Fran had told her not to eat bananas and grapes. Jo is concerned that Fran is giving incorrect dietary advice and patients are getting confused. She feels annoyed with Fran and wants to put her right but is anxious that Fran will get defensive and aggressive towards her. Like Tina she would like to be able to express her concerns clearly and calmly, to feel at ease with Fran and to gain her co-operation.

Although their situations are different each dietitian has similar thoughts and feelings. They all want their respective conversations to be a more rewarding experience than in the past. For this to happen, each needs first to be clear about the outcome they want. Ideally Nicky wants reassurance that she fulfilled her part, that her patient is not worse as a result of not getting the feeds and he will be given the supplements in future. Tina would like the GP to agree to use the diet sheets she has available. Jo would like Fran to give the same advice as she does. Being aware of their own thoughts and feelings and knowing what outcome they would like means they are each in a stronger position to communicate what they want assertively.

Developing assertiveness

Assertiveness means different things to different people and many are confused between assertiveness and aggression. Behaving assertively involves recognising our needs, expressing our thoughts and feelings, asking for what we want and listening to the other person. Being assertive is about being open and honest and communicating directly to the person concerned. When we behave assertively we are expressing an attitude of respect and acceptance of ourselves and the other person. We are acknowledging ourselves and others as human beings, each with qualities and frailties and each having a right to their unique view of the world. Speaking to be heard rather than speaking to be right is far from easy. We are constantly limited by our lack of perceptiveness, our fear of being in the wrong, our patterns of behaviour, and our social and cultural conditioning.

We are able to behave assertively when our self-esteem is high, when we value and accept ourselves – in other words when we perceive ourselves as 'I'm OK' and others as 'you're OK' (Berne 1970). This is a difficult attitude to maintain in an institution based on hierarchies such as the National Health Service (NHS), where one position in the organisation is seen as superior or inferior to another. This makes it difficult for staff to communicate honestly and directly with one another. On the one hand it is safer and more comforting to complain to a third party and evoke their sympathy than to risk the discomfort and uncertain consequences of confronting the person concerned. On the other hand the change we desire does not then take place. However, when we perceive ourselves and others as being neither superior nor inferior but as unique individuals, all with a valuable and different part to play, we are more likely to engage in open communication. As a result, changes are more likely to occur. Many people mistakenly think that those who are assertive are always calm and confident and do not feel angry or frightened. Anger, fear, nervousness and anxiety are emotions which we can communicate assertively, passively, manipulatively or aggressively. We are more able to behave assertively when the intensity of feeling is low. As emotions accumulate their intensity builds, discomfort increases and we express how we feel indirectly through manipulation or explosively through aggressive behaviour. Those who value their self-esteem will place great importance on acknowledging their feelings appropriately at an early stage when the level of feeling is manageable and acceptable for them.

In understanding assertiveness, it is useful to compare assertiveness with other ways of behaving, such as aggressiveness, passivity and manipulation.

Aggression

Aggression is about winning and getting our own way. When we think, 'You should . . .' and 'If I were you I'd do it this way' we are likely to feel frustrated and behave aggressively. Self-esteem is low and we attempt to feel better about ourselves by attacking and belittling the thoughts, values and capabilities of someone else. Aggression can be conveyed in low tones as well as raised voices. Other non-verbal signs may be obvious (shaking a fist) or subtle (pursing the lips). Often we may not think we are being aggressive and are surprised when we learn that we have been perceived that way. The resentment we have felt, but think we have successfully suppressed, leaks out through our communication.

Passivity

Passivity is about protecting ourselves and avoiding conflict and responsibility. When we behave passively we are anxious to please and willing to fit in with another at the expense of our own needs. However, we also lay ourselves open to being used and abused. When someone feels powerless and thinks of themselves as a victim of others or of their circumstances, and turns their anger inwards by blaming themselves, they behave passively. They may think, 'It's all my fault. If only I'd . . .'. At other times they may explode aggressively with 'It's all your fault, if only you had . . .'. Either way they maintain their low self-esteem and risk depression.

Manipulation

Manipulation uses techniques of persuasion, deviousness and cunning to get another to behave in a certain way. Often this is done in the form of a threat, for example, 'if you don't lose weight you'll become more and more disabled'. A situation is presented as being for the good of the other person. In denying the other person their right or ability to choose for themselves, the manipulative person is expressing a need to control another.

Steps towards becoming more assertive

No-one uses one form of behaviour exclusively. We react differently in different situations (Exercise 14.2). Behaving assertively increases the options for handling different situations. We experience having more personal power when we have more options. Becoming more assertive is a developmental process and does not happen as a result of attending a course or reading a book. Training courses and books provide foundations and information on which to build, but it is through continual practice, self-assessment and ongoing support that lasting change takes place.

Exercise 14.2

Notice how you behave in different situations. Make a note of when you would like to be more assertive. Start by being aware of how you behave. Is this passively, aggressively or manipulatively?

Prepare to behave assertively by being clear about what you want to say, how you feel and the outcome that you want. You can do this by asking yourself the following questions:

- Who is it I want to talk to?
- What do I want to say?
- How do I want to say it?
- When do I want to say it?
- Where do I want the communication to take place?
- What effect do I want to produce?
- What do I want to happen as a result?

Practise behaving assertively by:

- writing down what you want to say;
- making sure your message is specific and not long-winded;
- including how you feel and what you think;
- speaking for yourself using 'I', e.g. I think . . . , I feel . . . ;
- visualising yourself delivering your message effectively;
- rehearsing with someone with whom you feel safe.

Deliver your message assertively by:

- speaking clearly, audibly and firmly;
- maintaining eye contact and an open body posture;
- focusing on keeping calm and relaxed.

Listen to the response by:

- hearing what the other person says;
- reflecting to them to demonstrate that you have heard and to clarify your understanding;

- being prepared to repeat your assertion or to give another if this is appropriate.

The following situation is an example of a dietitian applying these skills when asking her manager for annual leave.

MANAGER: (*aggressively*) I can't have more than one of you off at the same time. Pat has already asked me for that week.

DIETITIAN: (*reflecting what has been said*) I understand that Pat has asked for that week, and that ideally you would prefer only one of us to be away. (*stating her position*) My problem is that I've been offered a place on a course I applied for. I've only just heard it's available now because someone has cancelled.

MANAGER: Well that's really inconvenient. I suppose you could ask Pat if she'll change but I really can't have both of you away at the same time.

DIETITIAN: (*maintaining her assertion*) I do want to do the course and feel disappointed about turning down this opportunity. I appreciate the timing is inconvenient. I will discuss it first with Pat as you suggest and then come back to you.

When first confronted we may feel surprise and react in a way which later we regret. For example, in the situation above the dietitian may behave passively saying meekly, 'That's OK. I won't go then' or manipulatively by saying 'Oh if Pat's already got that week I'll just have to turn down the offer'. In either case she is likely to feel resentful and her manager more annoyed.

Exercise 14.3

Read again the difficult situations for Nicky, Tina and Jo described earlier in this chapter. Now think how each could express themselves assertively by applying the guidelines given above: Nicky to her patient and ward staff, Tina to the GP and Jo to the practice nurse. It can be helpful to do the exercise with a partner so that you can compare notes and role play the scenarios. The aim of the person being Nicky, Tina or Jo is to maintain assertive behaviour for as long as they are able to during the conversation.

Giving criticism and praise

Some people give criticism without first considering the effect their remarks may have on others. Others feel so uncomfortable with the idea of having to criticise someone they hesitate to give it and spend time planning what to say so that the other person will not be upset.

They may hesitate so long that their feelings become too strong to contain. Then when they do speak their communication is aggressive, as in the following example of a dietitian saying impatiently to a student 'You should do it as you were shown the first time'. Later, and with more exasperation she says 'You still haven't got it right'.

Both remarks are examples of criticisms which blame the other person and so are likely to produce a defensive response. A dietitian behaving assertively would be more likely to say: 'I am concerned that you may not fully understand how to do it' followed by 'I think it would be a good idea if we went through the procedure again'. Although the student may feel upset these remarks are more likely to be received and accepted as feedback to be considered and acted on. The dietitian is conveying an attitude of imparting information to be heard rather than a desire to attach blame. Dietitians wanting to respond assertively find it useful to express what they want to say by constructing a sentence based on:

- *What I observe*, followed by a phrase describing the situation, e.g. 'I notice the medical notes are not available'.

Or if more appropriate:

- *What I hear the other person say*, e.g. 'When you tell me the medical notes aren't available . . .'.

Followed by:

- *How I feel*, e.g. 'I feel concerned', 'I feel frustrated'.
- *What I think*, e.g. 'I think it's important I read them before I see the patient'.
- *What I want/would like*, followed by the outcome they desire, e.g. 'I want to know how I can get hold of them' or 'I would like to get hold of them straight away'.

When this structure is followed, the remark is specific, open and honest. The phrase 'When (you) . . . I feel/I think . . .' is effective in both stating the facts as you perceive them and expressing how you feel or what you think about the situation and can be usefully used to give praise or offer compliments. For example, when a dietitian says to a student 'When you gave your talk on diet and renal disease I thought you presented the information very clearly'. When the sentence includes summarising or paraphrasing what the other person has just said it also acknowledges their difficulties, which gives scope for further exploration of the problem. For example, a dietitian, responding to a student who has not handed in a piece of work, says: 'When you tell me about your difficulties at home I realise why you have found it difficult to get your work done on time. I want to have marked all the essays by the end of the week. When can you let me have yours?'

The more able we are to give feedback which is specific, concise and acknowledges those concerned, the more fulfilling our experience. Communicating more openly and honestly requires that the dietitian remains non-defensive. She therefore needs to learn how to protect herself and behave assertively, as distinct from defending herself and behaving aggressively, passively or manipulatively.

Receiving criticism and praise

When we think we are being criticised and feel hurt, afraid, anxious, angry and confused, we can protect ourselves by behaving assertively. We usually deal with criticism by denying it, so avoiding it, or retorting and attacking back – in other words behaving passively or aggressively.

We can respond to criticism assertively by:

- asking for clarification (if we feel confused or unsure what the criticism is about);
- saying 'I will give the matter some thought' (if we feel overwhelmed and need time to consider the position);
- acknowledging the truth in the criticism (if it is partly true) and stating our assessment of the situation;
- agreeing (if the criticism is true);
- asserting that the criticism is unwarranted (if it is not true).

The following example of a dietitian and colleague compiling a data sheet together shows the dietitian responding in each of the ways described above. In reality she would use the one which is accurate for the occasion.

COLLEAGUE: You can't put that, it doesn't make sense.
DIETITIAN: (*asks for clarification*) It doesn't make sense to you?
or
DIETITIAN: (*needs time to consider*) I am surprised when you say it doesn't make sense. I need a bit of time to think about it.
or
DIETITIAN: (*acknowledges it is partly true and states her assessment*) Maybe it is a bit long-winded. I think we could rewrite this whole section.
or
DIETITIAN: (*calmly agrees with the truth*) Yes, I agree. Let's think of another way of putting it.
or
DIETITIAN: (*asserts the criticism is unwarranted*) I don't agree. It makes sense to me.

Exercise 14.4

Recall a time when you were criticised. Write down what was said and how you felt. Now write down your assertive response using one of the five ways as described in the text. Repeat this to yourself until you feel comfortable with it. Practise with a partner, asking them to say the criticism to you first. Then respond with your assertion. For the purpose of practice it is useful to formulate a response using all five ways, as in the example above.

It is often effective to include how we feel when we respond to a criticism, as in the following example: 'When you say, "You can't put that, it doesn't make sense", I want to react as though I'm under attack. I then want to stop working on this together. When I think about it calmly though I agree that there are ways in which it could be clearer.'

The phrase 'When you . . . I feel/think . . .' is also effective in both stating the facts as you perceive them and expressing how you feel about the situation. It can also be useful when acknowledging praise. Many find it difficult to accept praise or compliments without brushing the remark aside or denying it. For example 'When you tell me you enjoyed my presentation I feel encouraged' is a specific, honest and open acknowledgement of a dietitian's reaction to a compliment given by a colleague. Another effective way to respond to praise is to say a simple 'Thank you' which acknowledges that you have received the message. Brushing it aside, saying 'Oh it was nothing really', is likely to evoke a thought along the lines of 'I might as well not have bothered to say anything' and is experienced as a rejection.

It is important to focus on keeping calm if we are to maintain assertive behaviour in the face of another's non-assertiveness, for example when we are faced with someone who is behaving aggressively. Afterwards we may feel upset, hurt or angry and this is when it is valuable to focus on building self-esteem (Chapter 15).

Dealing with aggressive behaviour

When someone behaves aggressively towards us we frequently feel surprise, shock, fear and even panic. Having a strategy to follow is useful at such times. This section includes guidelines on three aspects: assessing the risk, defusing the situation and coping with the after-effects.

Assessing risks

It is useful to assess your job in terms of the following four headings:

(1) *What I do* – what aspects of my job may lead to people feeling annoyed, frustrated or afraid?
(2) *Who I'm with* – are there any particular groups or individuals who may be prone to unpredictable or aggressive behaviour?
(3) *Where I go* – do I work in any places that may carry an increased risk, e.g. making home visits?
(4) *When I am at risk* – are there certain times that are less safe than others?

Taking care of yourself

Important points to consider are:

- Noticing body language – look out for signs of restlessness, e.g. tapping feet, sighing.
- Being aware of factors which may irritate or annoy some people, e.g. being kept waiting.
- Trusting your intuition. Do you feel safe? If not remember your first priority is to keep yourself safe and act accordingly.
- Planning an escape route – is your exit blocked by anything, e.g. a chair or desk?
- Getting assistance if you need it, e.g. using panic buttons, mobile phones or creating a disturbance. Be specific when shouting for help, e.g. 'Help – call the police'.
- Being traceable if going elsewhere – letting someone know when and where you are going/due back and leaving details with someone.
- Knowing exactly where you are going and how to get there and if appropriate, where to park.
- Making home visits – when on the doorstep assess the situation and if in doubt, leave or arrange a time to call again with a colleague.
- Reporting any aggressive behaviour. Keeping it to yourself is no help to you or anyone else.

Defusing the situation

In the event of aggressive behaviour the following mnemonic (Be A DEFUSER) provides useful guidelines on how to defuse the situation.

Be A DEFUSER

Breathe – Focusing for a few seconds on your breathing will help you to keep calm.

*A*nticipate – Preparing yourself for what may happen next. If you suspect someone may use physical force towards you make it very clear straight away that this is unacceptable behaviour. For example you could say, 'I'm concerned that you may find it difficult to control your feelings. I want you to know that you are welcome to talk about how you feel but not to behave violently towards yourself, towards me or anything in this room.' If someone raises their voice to an unacceptable level an effective response is to state your limits, for example 'I am not willing to listen to you when you shout so loudly' or 'If you continue to shout I will leave this meeting'. Once limits are set in this way it is important that you are prepared to take the action you have specified and if necessary seek help.

*D*istance – considering how standing too close or moving forward increases intimidation.

*E*ye contact – maintaining this without glaring.

*F*ace the other person – not turning your back. If you need to get away move slowly backwards towards your escape route, keep talking and maintain eye contact whenever possible.

*U*se non-aggressive body language – be aware of both your own and that of the other person.

*S*peak slowly and clearly in a level tone.

*E*ncourage compromise – exploring possibilities, alternatives and options such as speaking to someone else about the situation instead of attempting to prove your point.

*R*eflect – focus on using your skills of active listening (Chapter 5) and reflective responding (Chapter 6).

Coping with the after-effects

After any incident which involves aggression or violence we are likely to experience shock and some form of stress-related response (Chapter 15). This is a normal reaction although the way we respond may be unique and depends on our general stress level and the seriousness of the incident. Possible reactions are:

- nausea;
- headaches;
- over/under sleeping or eating or drinking;
- feelings of anger, guilt or fear;
- reliving the situation either as daytime fantasy or nightmare;
- thinking 'I'm O.K. I can deal with this on my own'.

It is important to report all incidents no matter how insignificant they appear. Having the opportunity to speak about what happened from our point of view usually brings relief. This can take the form of managers or colleagues providing a 'listening ear' and practical support. It may involve calling on a professionally trained counsellor. By carefully and accurately assessing what happened and what changes could be made, the risk of future incidents can be reduced. We can cope more effectively both during and after an incident by managing our stress. The more practised we are in following techniques and strategies for managing stress the faster we are able to unwind after a stressful experience. The following are commonly accepted strategies:

- Taking regular exercise, eating healthily, developing self-awareness.
- Managing our time so as to have enough rest.
- Using techniques for relaxation and meditation.
- Having opportunities for self-expression and leisure.
- Building support with others through a variety of different relationships.

When these ways of managing stress become part of one's life they are readily accessible as a resource to call upon in times of need. The person whose stress level is high on a daily basis will take longer to unwind. Chapter 15 covers more on these topics.

Exercise 14.5

Think of a situation in which you have felt unsafe either physically or as a result of an aggressive verbal response. Consider the following questions:

(1)   What was it about the situation that was difficult or threatening?
(2)   What do you think caused it?
(3)   Do you think you or your colleagues may have contributed in any way to causing the incident? If so how?
(4)   What effect did the incident have on you (and your colleagues) both immediately and later? How did you feel?
(5)   How was the incident handled afterwards by either colleagues and/or your management?
(6)   How do you think the incident could have been better handled?

   This exercise can either be done on your own or with a partner when each of you take it in turns to ask the questions. The questioner needs to give enough time between questions for the other person to consider their response; also to use their skills of listening and responding in a supportive way (Chapters 5 and 6).

An ABC for handling confrontations

This alphabetical list has been designed to provide an easy reference for recalling the main points of effective confrontation.

Assumptions – check for any you might be making and minimise them by sticking to facts.

Behaviour – focus on the specific recent behaviour you want someone to change.

Core conditions (described in Chapter 3) – you will be more able to provide these when you are calm and relaxed.

Direct – confront the person concerned rather than a third party.

Empathy – demonstrate this by reflective responding (Chapter 6).

Feedback – state your observations of the facts as you perceive them.

Genuineness – be honest with yourself and prepared to share your thinking and feeling.

Have respect – for yourself and the other person.

I – speak for yourself by starting sentences with 'I think/feel/notice/hear . . .'.

Judgements – beware of these turning your feedback into criticism in which you are blaming another.

Keep calm – focus on this and delay any confrontation until you feel less stressed.

Language – avoid swearing and jargon.

Mirroring – create rapport by mirroring non-verbal communication. This helps you and the other person to listen attentively.

Nurture – take care of yourself when you are confronted and feel attacked.

Open mind – developing this enables you to be flexible and aware.

Perception – remember that yours may be different from that of another and that both are real to those concerned.

Questions – are confronting. Closed questions pose a higher risk of creating a barrier to further communication than open ones. Repeated questioning is intrusive and the receiver likely to react defensively.

Reflective responding – demonstrates that you have understood what has been said.

State facts – as you see them, e.g. 'This is how I see it . . .' or 'I think that . . .' and be prepared to include new facts as these come to light.

Take time – prepare yourself and take time to remain calm and focused. Give the other person time to assimilate what you have said.

Update – by assessing your handling of a confrontation and learning from each experience.

Voice – your voice reflects your attitude. Tune into and listen to yourself. Notice whether you are doing this as a way of informing, criticising or blaming yourself.

Watch – for non-verbal clues and be aware of incongruities.

eXpress – yourself clearly and concisely.

You – are the key to the way you handle the situation.

Zeal – and commitment to your development as a person will strengthen you in handling confrontations.

In this chapter ways of communicating assertively in dealing with difficult situations have been explored. The next chapter examines how the dietitian can obtain support for herself to help her in applying her counselling skills, as well as being able to deal with the difficult situations she may come across.

References

Berne, E. (1970) *Games People Play*. Penguin, London.
Dickson, A. (2004) *Difficult Conversations*. Piatkus Ltd, London.

Chapter 15

Support for the Dietitian

'Resolve to be thyself and know that he who finds himself, loses his misery'

Matthew Arnold

In this chapter I discuss:

- Knowing your limits
- Building self-esteem
- Coping with stress
- Building support
- About counselling
- Support from colleagues

Knowing your limits

Using counselling skills makes emotional demands of the dietitian which she may find difficult. When a dietitian is working effectively at this level with a patient she will find her own emotions aroused. As a result, she may find herself struggling with personal thoughts, feelings and situations with which she needs support and understanding. It is not only in a helping capacity that the dietitian can feel out of her depth in this way. There may be times with colleagues, those from other disciplines and managers, as well as in her personal life, when she experiences difficulties. To be truly effective in using counselling skills, she needs adequate training and ongoing skilled supervision to be an integral part of her work. The dietitian who feels supported in this way develops self-esteem and self-confidence and a willingness to take on more challenges and provide support for colleagues.

Beginning with self-assessment, this chapter explores ways in which the dietitian can gain support for herself and in so doing gain greater personal fulfillment. Working within her limits while continually developing these through ongoing learning, is a challenge for the dietitian using counselling skills. Exercise 15.1 is designed to help the reader become more aware of her limits as a skilled helper.

Exercise 15.1

Think of a time with a patient when you thought you were out of your depth. Reflect on each question and make notes for yourself.

(1)   What led me to feeling doubtful about my ability to help this patient? This could be (i) something to do with dietetics, (ii) something the patient said or did, or (iii) something personal for you.
(2)   Is this an isolated example or am I generally lacking in confidence?
(3)   How did my thoughts and feelings affect the way I was with this patient?
(4)   How do I feel, and what thoughts come to mind, about seeing them again?
(5)   If I were to see this patient on another occasion or to have more time with them, could I help them effectively?
(6)   Do I think this person needs help in a specialist area?

The questions can be adapted to apply to different situations and other people, for example meetings with colleagues. Your notes can be a useful basis for discussion in a supervisory or counselling session.

In the following example Jan, a basic-grade dietitian, has been told that next month she will be expected to cover three extra wards in addition to her own while a colleague is away. She is worried she will not be able to manage and that the service to patients will deteriorate. She adapts the points given in Exercise 15.1, and asks herself the following questions, making a note of the thoughts that then occur to her:

Q: What has led me to feeling so worried? Is it because I don't think I can do the work?
A: I'm doing it anyway – it's just there will be more of it.
Q: Is it something about the way the new plan was put to me?
A: The first time it was mentioned was when I was in the office with Ann (*a colleague*) and she mentioned she was going to be away. Then Carol (*the manager*) phoned and told me about the arrangements she had made to cover for Ann which included me taking on the extra wards.
Q: How confident have I been feeling lately?

A: I have been feeling OK. Now I've got on top of the work it's not demanding at all. In fact I've been thinking lately that I could do with a change!

Q: How did my thoughts and feelings affect the way I was with both Ann and Carol?

A: I feel envious of Ann for being able to take time off and angry with Carol for making the arrangements without consulting me. I haven't wanted to have anything to do with either of them since!

Having thought about these questions and her answers, Jan realises that her anxiety is not so much about her lack of confidence in doing the job but more to do with the way this change in her workload was presented to her. She acknowledges she wants some time off herself; also that she wants to accept the challenge of taking on the new wards. She feels relieved that her confidence in her ability to do the work is restored. She also has a hunch that she has learned something important about herself to do with feeling angry and then becoming filled with self-doubt. She decides she needs more time to think about this. She also realises that increasing her workload is placing greater demands on herself and she wonders what extra support she could have. Maybe regular meetings with senior colleagues, opportunities to give feedback to her manager and plans for a holiday for herself will help. She decides to discuss the details about handing over her work with Ann and to ask Carol about annual leave and support while taking on the extra work.

Building self-esteem

The way in which the dietitian thinks and feels about herself is crucial to her ability to be assertive (Chapter 14). When she feels a sense of well-being and is satisfied with life, she experiences herself and those around her as worthwhile human beings. In transactional analysis (TA) this is known as 'I'm OK you're OK' (Berne 1970). Our attitude shifts when we are not satisfied, when we think and feel that life could be different in some way. We may think of ourselves as 'I'm OK' and others as 'You're not OK' or 'I'm not OK but you're OK'. When we feel despairing we adopt a position of 'I'm not OK you're not OK'. These positions are known as life positions and we each have one that is fundamental to us. Life positions are defined as one's basic belief formed in childhood, about oneself and others, which is used to justify decisions and behaviour (Stewart & Joines 1987). In adult life we shift from one position to another throughout the day (Exercise 15.2).

Life positions

I'm OK, you're OK
I'm OK, you're not OK
I'm not OK, you're OK
I'm not OK, you're not OK

T.A. Harris (1995)

Exercise 15.2

Think about yourself in relation to the four life positions described above. Which one are you adopting now? Reflect on your day and be aware when you were in a different position. What was happening then? In what circumstances are you likely to change position? How might you think and feel in each position? What might you say and do?

Self-awareness

Self-esteem is increased by developing self-awareness. However, becoming aware of the way in which we think, feel and behave can result in becoming temporarily more self-critical. When we develop the detachment whereby we can suspend judgement, we are able to observe ourselves in each of the life positions, and learn how we can spend more time in the healthy position which is fundamental to building self-esteem.

There are many ways in which we can develop our awareness. One way is giving ourselves time to reflect, time to relax and time for ourselves. This is not easy for many who find themselves rushing to do more and more to meet the demands of work, family and friends, which leaves little time to meet their own needs. Frantic as we may feel at times, it can be more comfortable initially to continue in this cycle of activity than to step aside and explore how to make changes. Many of us value the belief that we should put others first and we consider it selfish to think of ourselves and our needs. However, to habitually put the needs of others before our own is to deny ourselves. In not meeting our own needs we develop a dependence on others to do this for us. When they fail to do so we can become resentful towards them and may conclude that they are ignorant, uncaring and selfish.

By increasing our self-awareness we can learn what it is we want or need at any particular time. Using our ability to be assertive we can openly and honestly share this with another (Exercise 15.3). We can enhance our self-esteem by learning to acknowledge and give to ourselves what we most want.

Exercise 15.3

Spend a few minutes thinking of something you want right now. This may be something which would help you to feel more comfortable physically, such as a rest, or emotionally, such as talking to someone, or mentally, such as something which stimulates and distracts you. Jot down whatever comes to mind. Be specific, e.g. I want ten minutes with no interruptions so that I can finish this report. Pick one of the items and imagine yourself asking for this passively, aggressively, manipulatively and assertively (see example below). Notice the different words you use, the changes in your non-verbal communication and how you feel.

Examples of different responses to an unwanted interruption:

'It doesn't matter. I can do this later'. (*Passive*)
'Go away. I can't see you now.' (*Aggressive*)
'Can't you see I'm busy!' (*Manipulative*)
'Unfortunately now is not a good time to talk as I need to finish this report.' (*Assertive*)

Acknowledgement

Most of us can recall painful moments when we have been ignored, when we have not had our thoughts, feelings or behaviour acknowledged. When this happens we feel disappointed and undervalued and may respond by withdrawing into ourselves or behaving more outrageously in an attempt to get the attention we need. In short, our self-esteem is lowered.

Being able to give and receive acknowledgement openly and genuinely raises self-esteem. Acknowledgement is a recognition of the existence of someone or something, of feelings and behaviour or of how things are or have been. One of our basic needs is to be recognised and acknowledged, and giving acknowledgement is a supportive intervention when concerned with helping others (Heron 2001). Acknowledgement can be confused with praise. We may praise someone or something because we think this is what is expected of us or because we want to encourage someone, rather than because we genuinely mean it. The effect of praising someone can be to lower self-esteem and create dependency or resentment. When praise is given as a generalised 'Well done' the recipient may think they have been patronised and feel angry and resentful. On the other hand they may feel pleased and grateful and encouraged to seek further approval. Praise is the opposite of criticism (Chapter 14) and both are ways in which we express our judgements and opinions. An acknowledgement is a statement of what is, a recognition of the existence of something or somebody. Acknowledgement is neither good nor bad. In other words it does not include a value judgement.

The more we can genuinely and honestly acknowledge ourselves, the more we can express ourselves honestly and appropriately with others and in so doing raise self-esteem. Many find keeping a private journal a useful way to begin the process of honestly acknowledging their thoughts and feelings and an ideal way of taking care of our emotional well-being, of working through decisions, of recording fears and triumphs. Keeping a journal provides a rehearsal space to bring together thoughts, ideas and emotions before revealing them to others (Waines 2004).

Acknowledging achievements on a daily basis is a way to develop self-esteem. Acknowledging events which we consider mistakes or failures is to acknowledge our disappointments and frustrations. When we can do this with the intention of learning from the experience, instead of admonishing or reprimanding oneself, we become more honest, genuine and open to ourselves. Doing this on a monthly and annual basis is an effective way of reviewing and assessing oneself.

Exercise 15.4

Take a few minutes to consciously relax. Then write down your achievements of the day. Be sure to include those you consider too small to count, e.g. getting to work on time. Be aware of your thoughts and feelings about doing this exercise. Notice if you find it easier to focus on lack of achievement.

Tips for building self-esteem

The following tips are useful both for the dietitian herself and for her to discuss with patients who want to build their self-worth.

- Take time for yourself. (*This can be difficult for many people to do.*)
- Give yourself a treat every day whether you think you deserve it or not. (*It could be useful to discuss the significance of food or alcohol as a treat with patients.*)
- Make a note of your achievements. (*Of the day, the week, the month, the year and your life!*)
- Give yourself the rest you need. This may involve altering your habit of going to bed late or forcing yourself to work when you are unwell.

- Express appreciation of yourself and someone else.
- Develop a stronger sense of personal direction. Set goals for yourself. (*It is useful to discuss the thoughts and feelings associated with failing to meet these.*)
- Take a risk each day – one which extends yourself beyond your comfort zone. (*New experiences, however small, raise our energy.*)
- Take care of yourself. Act in ways which will ensure no harm to yourself or another.
- Seek out and ask for support when you want it.
- Accept responsibility for your own actions. (*When speaking, notice the difference when 'I' is used instead of 'you'.*) Be aware when you blame another. In trying to get another to take responsibility you disempower yourself.
- Be patient, kind and gentle with yourself.

Coping with stress

Although stress has a negative connotation, it is a fact of life that we need a certain amount of stress to function effectively. The flight or fight response we experience in response to impending danger enables us to flee or perform heroic feats in the face of seemingly insurmountable tasks. A certain level of stress is necessary in order to give a rewarding performance. Stress becomes negative, however, when we feel out of control and think we are exceeding our ability to cope. When this happens excitement and anticipation become anxiety and fear. We realise there is a gap between how we want life to be and how life actually is at present.

We can feel stressed as a result of too much or too little stimulation. This stimulation can be internal – such as a lack of fulfilment, an unresolved conflict or a past memory – or it can be external, such as a major life change or an environmental stress, for example noise or pollution. It is well recognised that the process of change creates stress and certain events in our lives induce more stressful reactions than others. Stress is associated with, and contributes to, some physical conditions and there is evidence of the influence of stress on the immune system and physical illness (Greener 2002).

The quicker we can unwind the less opportunity there is for the cumulative effect to develop. We develop various strategies for coping with stress, some of which are more healthy than others. In learning to manage stress so that we minimise the harmful effects, we can begin to take charge of ourselves, our self-esteem rises and our ability to assert ourselves increases. We begin to function more effectively and our stress level subsides. Managing stress becomes a priority if we are to help others and ourselves.

Stress affects us both physically and mentally. The first step in managing stress is to assess our own level of stress and become aware of how we are affected by different situations (Exercise 15.5). Knowing this we can build up a variety of ways to unwind.

Exercise 15.5

The following questions are designed to increase your understanding of your own stress. Tick the questions to which you answer yes. Although the exercise is not a validated tool for measuring stress, the answers provide a guide to your personal degree of stress.

- Do you often hurry when you don't have to?
- Are you often distracted or preoccupied by your thoughts while supposedly listening to someone else?
- When you have a problem which you can't deal with until later, do you spend time worrying about it now?
- Are you finding it difficult to express your feelings or confide in those with whom you have a close relationship?
- Do you face problems irritably and get excited easily?
- Does your heart feel like it is pounding during normal activities?
- Do you feel constant dryness in your throat and mouth?
- Are you prone to impulsive behaviour?
- Do your emotions run up and down the scale easily?
- Do you sometimes feel the overwhelming urge to cry or run away and hide?
- Do you find you are unable to concentrate on the task at hand?
- Do you bump into things in your effort to get from place to place?
- Do you feel accident prone lately?
- Do you experience feelings of unreality, weakness or dizziness?
- Do you feel tired all the time with little excitement about life?
- Are you easily startled by small sounds?
- When you hear yourself laughing is it high pitched and nervous?
- Do you tremble or have nervous tics in your facial muscles?
- Do you feel afraid of something but don't know what it is?
- Do you move about restlessly and find it difficult to settle?
- Do you feel queasy, have indigestion, vomiting or diarrhoea?
- Do you have nagging pains in your back, neck or shoulders?
- Have you been getting migraine headaches?
- Have you lost your appetite or are you having bouts of excessive hunger?
- Have you increased your use of medicines?
- Have you increased your use of alcohol?
- Do you take tranquillisers on a regular basis?

- Do you have nightmares or wake feeling exhausted?
- Do you feel more anxious than content?
- Do you wake sporadically?

If you have answered yes to more than half the questions stress is becoming an issue and you could be on the way to developing levels that are too high. If you answered no to all the questions you probably weren't being honest. Most of us tend to underestimate our own stress levels.

Ways to unwind

There are several actions we can take on a mental and physical level which are useful in reducing stress. Engaging in an activity such as clearing out a cupboard, for example, may regain a sense of control, and physical activity such as dancing or swimming can provide release from tension held in the body. A simple and effective exercise which is less strenuous is to focus on breathing for a few minutes when stressed. This calms any thoughts which keep occurring.

Our attitude also affects the way we handle stressful situations. If we are in the position of 'I'm not OK' (see earlier in this chapter) we can help ourselves by taking steps to build our self-esteem. If we are in the position of 'I'm OK, you're not OK' we can help ourselves by examining what it is we think 'not OK' about the other person and consider how we can express our thoughts and feelings towards them in an assertive rather than aggressive way.

Talking to someone is the action many would choose, yet if the person we talk to is not able to listen effectively we may regret having spoken. Many find writing helps gain perspective and understanding about a problem or a difficult situation. Others find that listing practical options presented by a problem, choosing one and acting on it, helps them to feel more in charge of a situation. On the other hand delaying action by setting the problem on one side for a while and becoming engrossed in something else is a useful way to give oneself time. Developing the knack of shrugging off worries, literally and mentally, can have the effect of setting them on one side for a while. However, this may not be a useful strategy for the person who habitually procrastinates to avoid dealing with something.

When thinking about a problem it is helpful to consider taking an opposite approach. One way to do this is to ask oneself questions such as: What if (the opposite) were the case? What do I think would happen? How might I feel? Picturing the worst that can happen can feel scary, yet exaggerating a situation and giving form to our worst fantasies allows us to consider if this is really likely to happen. Gaining a different perspective on a situation releases tension and results in greater understanding. Imagining a few years from now and asking how much it will matter then, has the effect of distancing us from a problem.

Humour also gives a different perspective on a situation. Being able to see a funny or ridiculous side can help us laugh off tension and release stress. Considering the good aspects of a difficult situation, of which there are always some despite our difficulty in realising these, gives a balanced view. We are then more able to see things in proportion and consider ways of resolving the difficulty. Imagining ourselves as being successful and feeling good about the situation, that is moving more into a position of 'I'm OK, you're OK' (see earlier in this chapter), is a healthy direction to aim for. The more we consider this to be our life position the more able we are to stop, pause and focus on the present instead of reliving the past or creating fantasies of the future.

As explained in Chapter 7 cognitive-behavioural therapy (CBT) can help us to change the way we think and perceive an event. We can learn to do this by changing the negative thoughts associated with stressful feelings. Exercise 15.6 is designed to help the reader with this and can be applied to any behaviour.

Exercise 15.6

Think of an example of something you find stressful, for example getting to work on time. Taking a sheet of paper head the first page 'My journey to work'. Make three separate columns heading one 'Action', one 'Thought' and one 'Feeling'. As you make your journey to work note in the appropriate column each of your actions, thoughts and feelings. Assess the intensity of the feeling you experience by assigning a number between 1 and 10. As you ask yourself how much you are experiencing this feeling note the first number which comes to mind as usually this is the most accurate. An example is given below.

Action	Thoughts	Feelings	Scale of feeling
Ran to bus stop	It'll be awful to miss it	Anxiety	7/10
Climbed on bus	Hurrah, I've got it	Relief	5/10
Stood for journey	This is no way to travel	Irritation	8/10
Got off bus	Thank goodness that's over	Relief	4/10

Look back over your comments and make a note of your observations.

In the illustration given above the thought 'It will be awful to miss it' when running to the bus stop is associated with a negative outcome. The intensity of the anxiety and the irritation felt later is greater than the intensity of the relief. If when running to the bus stop the thought had been 'I intend to catch this bus but if I don't it's not the end of the world', the perceived outcome would be positive and the associated feeling would be one of purposefulness. If the thought associated with standing for the journey were changed from 'This is no way to travel' to 'At least I'm on my way even though I've got to stand' the associated feeling is relief rather than irritation. In the example given, anxiety and irritation are felt more intensely than relief. However, changing the thoughts changes the balance and as a result other emotions (relief and purposefulness) are dominant. The reader is recommended to experiment with consciously reframing her thoughts and being aware of her feelings in a number of different situations. The following is an example of a dietitian practising this at a meeting with a consultant.

> Sarah waits for the consultant to finish talking to the doctors gathered around him. She thinks, 'This is a waste of time. Even though I arranged a time to see him and I am here on time he's never available. He'll be rushing off somewhere else in a minute.' She feels increasingly irritable and sighs, shifting her weight from one foot to the other. 'It's as though I don't matter', she concludes. Suddenly aware of this thought she feels shocked and consciously decides to reframe her thoughts. 'I matter to me. I believe that what I have to say is important and valuable. I have done my part and arranged this meeting. I am here as we agreed. He is busy and may have forgotten about his meeting with me. He may not have time to discuss matters with me now but whatever happens it is not a waste of my time because I am using it to help myself deal with this situation differently. I do have choices: I could interrupt him, I could go away and I could wait longer. I now need to weigh up the pros and cons of each option and decide upon one. I'm now feeling less hopeless and have more energy.'

Building support

Although we may be experiencing considerable stress we feel more able to cope when we know that we have another with whom to share our difficulties. When we feel supported we feel less alone. However, relying on one or two sources of support may place a burden on these people who may not be able to provide the amount or type of support we require. If our need is great our expectations are likely to be high and it will be more likely that another, however willing at first, will be unable to live up to our demands. Building a support network is a way of ensuring we are able to get the support we need from a number of sources (Exercise 15.7).

> **Exercise 15.7**
>
> Sit quietly and allow yourself to relax. Take a blank sheet of paper and place a mark or symbol in the centre to represent yourself. Think of the people in your life who you consider supportive of you. These may be friends, family, colleagues and anyone who provides you with a service, e.g. your doctor. Using a symbol which represent these people, e.g. their initials, place them in a position on the paper which reflects how you perceive them relative to yourself in the centre. Reflect on the position for each. What role do they fulfil? Have you a confidante among your supporters? Do you have someone with whom you feel wanted? Who can you turn to in an emergency? Who is a good resource for information? Will someone challenge you and give you honest feedback? With whom would you share sorrow or joy?
>
> As you answer these questions notice how many times the same name occurs. In what ways can you widen your support network, e.g. through social or professional groups?

Talking through a problem with someone who is able to listen fully (Chapters 5 and 6) can provide insights and clarity to deal with the problem in a new way. Dietitians who have colleagues with whom they can give and receive such support are in a valuable position. Talking to a counsellor is another way to obtain support which is different from seeking the advice and support of colleagues, friends and family. Some people think they need to be in desperate straits to warrant counselling. However, a crisis may be averted if someone has had the support and developed some resources through counselling to manage a difficult situation more effectively.

About counselling

An understanding of counselling is useful when discussing this form of support with patients. It is also useful for dietitians who choose to seek counselling as a form of support for themselves and for those who are considering formal training in counselling skills. The following description of counselling is adapted from information published by the British Association for Counselling and Psychotherapy (2006b):

> Counselling takes place when a counsellor sees a client in a private and confidential setting to explore a difficulty the client is having or distress they may be experiencing. Counselling is always at the request of the client. By

listening attentively the counsellor can begin to perceive the difficulties from the client's point of view. Counselling is a way of enabling choice, reducing confusion and helping someone to make changes.

The relationship takes place within agreed boundaries which may specify duration, regularity, availability and confidentiality. The counsellor's role is to facilitate the client's work in ways which respect the client's values, personal resources and capacity for self-determination.

Nowadays more and more people are seeking counselling and some ask if there is a difference between counselling and psychotherapy. After much debate the British Association for Counselling and Psychotherapy (2006b) has concluded that it is not possible to make a generally accepted distinction. In recent years there has been a rapid growth in the number of counsellors undergoing training and in the use of counselling services by organisations. Although there is a growing acceptance of counselling, there is still confusion and mystery about the process of counselling and the work that counsellors do. This leads many people to invest counsellors with powers they do not have and to fear the process that might occur if they were to have counselling for themselves. Some have the mistaken belief that a counsellor will solve their problems or at least tell them what they should do. Others are concerned that during counselling they may discover aspects of themselves that they would rather not know. People seek professional help when their desire for their life to be different is greater than their anxiety about counselling. Counselling can help with:

- reducing anxiety;
- easing depression and unhappiness;
- learning to trust again;
- increasing self-esteem and self-confidence;
- exploring problems;
- facing difficult decisions.

What does counselling involve?

The nature of counselling means that the counselling session is unpredictable as well as intense. Neither counsellor nor client know beforehand what will occur in their work together. This adventure into the unknown means that counselling has an immediacy that is exciting, rewarding and demanding. The immediacy increases with the counsellor's ability to empathise, accept and be genuine with the client, that is provide the therapeutic components of the counselling relationship identified by Rogers (1976). These are referred to in the person-centred tradition as the core conditions (Mearns & Thorne 1999) and are described in Chapter 3.

In order that counselling can take place, it is important for both client and counsellor that each has a clear understanding of the practical arrangements for working together. Such arrangements concern when they will meet, for how long, the fee involved, and provision for changing these agreements. Other issues which form part of the working agreement concern the nature and limitations of confidentiality and the changes that the client wants to make as a result of counselling. By establishing a contract in this way a framework is developed within which the intense, unpredictable and therapeutic nature of counselling can take place.

Who seeks counselling?

People of all ages and backgrounds may seek professional help at some time in their lives. Breakdown in relationships, bereavement or a stressful change in one's life may result in someone questioning their purpose, goals or meaning of life and may bring them into a counselling relationship.

Our psychological health is closely linked to our physical health, and inner conflicts may result in somatisation of stress and the development of a variety of physical ailments. Emotional problems do not just go away and although we may try to suppress our feelings they can leak out in the form of migraine headaches, backaches, low energy, tension, stress, temper outbursts and depression. These in turn can lead to behaviours such as smoking, binge-eating, excessive alcohol intake and drug taking which in turn can affect relationships, employment and family life.

Referral for counselling may come via a medical practitioner who recognises the link between mental and physical distress but many people refer themselves. Some do this by approaching recognised organisations who provide a counselling service, whereas others make their own arrangements by looking in directories which list individual counsellors. Many find a counsellor through personal recommendation.

Clients come to counselling with varying degrees of self-awareness and clarity about what they want to focus on and what they want from the counsellor. Their needs can be grouped under six broad headings:

- Developmental

The focus is on individual growth and development, for example the client who wants to gain self-confidence.

- Problem focused

The client wants help to cope with a particular problem.

- Decision making

The client wants help in making a specific decision.

- Crisis

The client's resources to cope are under great stress.

- Following trauma

A client is helped to recover from a deeply shocking experience that occurred some time in the past.

- Support

This helps a client develop and use their own resources.

Training in counselling

The British Association for Counselling and Psychotherapy is one of the main professional bodies for counsellors in Britain and represents members' interests on a wide range of issues including training. Their *Ethical Framework for Good Practice in Counselling and Psychotherapy* (2002) lays down guidelines on standards for both counselling practice and training.

Training courses available range from introductory to intermediate and advanced level, with the award of certificates, diplomas and degrees depending on the level of the course. Courses are mainly part-time and are frequently based on a modular system. The *Training in Counselling and Psychotherapy Directory* (British Association for Counselling and Psychotherapy 2006c) provides information on organisations offering training courses which are recognised by the British Association for Counselling and Psychotherapy. The directory is available from the organisation (contact details are given in Appendix 2).

An introductory course with a practical focus on counselling skills is useful as a first step for anyone wanting to find out if they wish to pursue further training. After completing an introductory course it is worth taking time to consider carefully the following points before pursuing further training:

- Do I want to become a professional counsellor or do I want to develop my skills to incorporate them more effectively in my work?
- What commitment do I want to make?

Training can be expensive. There are tuition fees, personal therapy and supervision fees, books and conference fees as well as extra training in personal development. Training involves a greater time commitment than might be anticipated from the tuition hours.

- What counselling orientation am I interested in?

There are many theories and models (Chapter 1). Some of these are based on ideas which are current at the time, whereas others are supported by much literature and research. Some courses integrate more than one model.

- How do I get to see clients?

Are the patients I see in my work suitable for the purposes of my course? Will I get sufficient experience this way? Am I prepared to do voluntary counselling for an agency?

- Am I prepared to be a client and have counselling for myself?

In order to be able to develop and use her skills with clients, a counsellor will have explored her own beliefs and attitudes in considerable depth. Counsellors are required to continually confront themselves, to learn how to question what previously they had accepted unquestioningly, and to develop their own philosophy.

Considering the many courses on offer and the commitment required in time, money and personal development, it is worth researching before registering on a particular course of training. An information sheet *Training and Careers in Counselling and Psychotherapy* has been published by the British Association for Counselling and Psychotherapy (2006a).

A personal perspective on working as a counsellor

Remaining person-centred with a client as they struggle to find an answer for themselves is not easy. Yet, as a client myself, I recall many occasions when being allowed the opportunity to do just that has been enriching for me. When I remember my own experiences I am encouraged to trust my clients' ability to help themselves, as well as the therapeutic effect of the relationship between us.

There are times when my ability to provide the core conditions for a client is deeply tested. The times when I find it most difficult to listen fully to a client are those times when I think I have the answer to their problem. There are also times when I do not find it easy to distinguish between the emotions which I feel in response to my client and those which are aroused as a result of my own personal experience. Providing an opportunity for a client to experience themselves in a new way is particularly rewarding. Being with a client when they gain a personal insight is enriching for me as well as for the client. Creating a relationship in which the client feels safe to express more of themselves enhances my personal development and I find that having a client trust me enough to share themselves openly and genuinely in my presence is a moving and humbling experience.

In endeavouring to provide the core conditions, I find personal therapy, supervision and the general support of friends and colleagues to be invaluable. Being able to talk through a problem with someone who is experienced in counselling provides me with support and greater understanding. A client's problem may closely relate to difficulties of my own and sometimes highlights for me an area to explore further in my own therapy. As I continue to learn to be more genuine, empathic and accepting of myself I am aware that I am also more able to bring these core conditions to my relationship with my clients.

Colleagues can also be a valuable support in providing opportunities for stimulating discussion. Membership of a professional counselling organisation provides me with access to continuing training and development and also meets my need to belong to a body with credibility and influence which represents my professional status. It is important to me to keep a balance in my life. Spending time with others and alone, and having opportunities to take part in physical and creative non-counselling related activities helps me to keep this balance.

Support from colleagues

Some areas in which dietitians may need support are often about:

- difficult situations concerning patients;
- the tasks they are expected to do;
- managing relationships within the department;
- negotiating and clarifying roles with members of their multidisciplinary team;
- carving a role for themselves within a team;
- the impact upon their work of emotional and practical issues at home;
- making decisions about their future career;
- managing their own health concerns.

Any and all of the above may occur at any time. A dietitian may experience stress in more than one area at a time. At such times she is likely to need considerable support. When several people who work together have training in counselling skills they can greatly support one another and others. An effective way to do this is to establish regular informal sessions in which they take it in turns to listen to each other.

The following guidelines are intended to help those wanting to engage in providing this form of mutual support. The guidelines underline the desirability for both people to keep clear boundaries.

Making arrangements

- Agree when to meet, for how long, e.g. 45 minutes, and how often, e.g. once a month.
- Decide where to meet bearing in mind you want privacy and freedom from distractions and interruptions.
- Decide how long you are going to meet for, e.g. 6 months, to be renewed if appropriate.
- Agree how you deal with issues of confidentiality and cancelling meetings.

Managing the session

- Agree how to divide the time, e.g. 15 minutes with five minutes to debrief allows 20 minutes each and with an extra five minutes to cover any practical issues such as a date for next time (= 45 minutes).
- Decide who is to be in the listening role first. The challenge for the listener is to maintain her focus on her colleague and not be diverted on to her own casework. This can easily happen with those working in the same profession. It can be helpful to both if the speaker declares at the beginning of her time what she would like to get from talking through her 'problem'.
- It is the listener's responsibility to keep the time and to draw the session to a close.
- The 'debriefing' time is an opportunity for each to share how they experienced the session.
- Be aware of the session breaking down into a two-way conversation. Remember it is an opportunity for each in turn to have time to be heard and understood by another.
- Be aware that this is not the time for gossip. It is a time to practise one's skills of active listening and to develop ongoing learning.
- It is not a substitute for skilled casework supervision but can be a mutually supportive addition.

Supervision

This term is familiar to counsellors for whom regular supervision is an essential requirement in order to practise as accredited counsellors. For many health professionals, supervision is seen as necessary for the inexperienced or incompetent rather than a means of providing necessary ongoing professional support and learning. Counsellors perceive supervision as a time to debrief, discuss work-related problems, gain information and emotional support. Dietitians who specialise in eating disorders and receive casework supervision usually find this valuable and beneficial. Dietitians who are considering lobbying for their own casework supervision may find the following points – adapted from an information sheet on supervision (British Association for Counselling and Psychotherapy 2000) – useful when developing their own guidelines.

- Counselling supervision is a formal arrangement for counsellors to discuss their work regularly with someone who is experienced in counselling and supervision.
- It is a process to maintain adequate standards of counselling and a method of consultancy to widen the horizons of the experienced counsellor.
- It is an opportunity to discuss in confidence the demands placed upon the counsellor.
- It can help the counsellor relate theory to practice and vice versa. Thus it is an aspect of ongoing training.
- The role of the supervisor is different from that of the line manager. A supervisor needs to have training in supervision and be a qualified and experienced counsellor.
- The precise nature of the supervisor's profession is less important than their skill in counselling and rapport with the counsellor concerned.
- Supervision can be on a one-to-one or group basis.

Making use of supervision – a dietitian's experience

For some time Jackie had felt in need of support in using counselling skills in her work. When she heard that there was an opportunity for her to have individual casework supervision she arranged to have a 45-minute session once a month. Although she knew the sessions were confidential, she felt nervous as the time for her first session got nearer because she was not sure how to make best use of the time. She recalled the patients she had seen in the last week and the interview with one in particular came to mind as she had found it difficult at the time.

The patient had broken down in tears almost as soon as she had arrived to see Jackie. 'Ah ha,' Jackie had thought 'This is where I use my counselling skills!' She had focused on giving her attention to the patient, acknowledging how upset her patient seemed and had invited her to talk about what was troubling her. Jackie had felt pleased that she had been able to do this calmly yet she had not been prepared for the long and involved story which the patient then told her. She had begun to feel overwhelmed and worried that she was not going to have time to focus on her patient's diet. She had hastily diverted the patient on to this by reassuring her that all would be all right in the end. She had covered all she meant to by the end of the interview but she was not sure the patient had understood her advice about the diet. Afterwards she had felt awkward and uncaring yet what else could she have done?

In her supervision session Jackie recounted the interview and explored different ways in which she could have ended on time more appropriately and less abruptly. She was able to understand more clearly how her patient's distress had affected her and led her to deal with the situation in the way she had. She left the session feeling more able to distinguish the difference between her role as a dietitian and her role as helpful listener. She decided to read about setting appropriate boundaries and to practise doing this more often (Chapters 4 and 13).

At her next session Jackie talked about an incident with a registrar on a ward round. Jackie had strongly advised a certain dietary modification and had been taken aback when the registrar had suddenly shouted at her in disagreement. She had not realised until later how distressed she felt as at the time she thought she had responded quite smartly. In supervision she explored what had happened using a model which was new to her. She realised how she could apply her new understanding in other interactions and modify her approach in similar situations.

At another session Jackie talked about her concerns about having students with her – how best to respond to them and her anxiety about being observed by someone else. She considered ways of applying her counselling skills with students and came away with a clearer idea of how she could provide effective support for the student and herself.

In a later session Jackie reviewed what she had learned in supervision. She outlined the situations she had brought to the sessions, the issues that she had explored, what she had learned and how she had made use of this in her work in a brief report. At first the idea of having 45 minutes set aside for her alone had seemed a luxury she could not justify. At times she had felt frustrated because there seemed no simple answers only more for her to think about yet she realised that far from being an indulgence the sessions were challenging work yet stimulating. Jackie concluded that she had found the sessions a valuable way of consolidating her learning about counselling skills and developing her knowledge. As a result of the support she had received she felt more supported herself and more able to offer support to others, as well as more confident, motivated and encouraged to continue using her skills.

References

Berne, E. (1970) *Games People Play*. Penguin, London.

British Association for Counselling and Psychotherapy (2000) *What is Supervision?* British Association for Counselling and Psychotherapy, Rugby.

British Association for Counselling and Psychotherapy (2002) *Ethical Framework for Good Practice in Counselling and Psychotherapy*. British Association for Counselling and Psychotherapy, Rugby.

British Association for Counselling and Psychotherapy (2006a) *Training and Careers in Counselling and Psychotherapy*. British Association for Counselling and Psychotherapy, Rugby.

British Association for Counselling and Psychotherapy (2006b) *What is Counselling?* British Association for Counselling and Psychotherapy, Rugby.

British Association for Counselling and Psychotherapy (2006c) *Training and Psychotherapy Resource Directory*. British Association for Counselling and Psychotherapy, Rugby.

Greener, M. (2002) *The Which? Guide to Managing Stress*. Which Ltd, London.

Harris, T.A. (1995) *I'm OK – You're OK*. Arrow Books Ltd, London.

Heron, J. (2001) *Helping the Client*, 5th edn. Sage Publications, London.

Mearns, D. & Thorne, B. (1999) *Person Centred Counselling in Action*. Sage Publications, London.

Rogers, C. (1976) *Client Centred Therapy*. Constable & Robinson, London.

Stewart, I. & Joines, V. (1987) *TA Today – A New Introduction to Transactional Analysis*. Lifespace Publishing, Nottingham.

Waines, A. (2004) *The Self Esteem Journal: Using a Journal to Build Self Esteem*. Sheldon Press, London.

Postscript

Summaries and points for discussion

The following brief summaries focus on the main points I have
attempted to communicate in the book. The questions which follow
each section are designed to raise issues for consideration and discussion. I trust both summaries and questions will be helpful to readers
when reflecting on what they have read.

Part 1   A counselling approach

Chapter 1 considers the traditional role of the dietitian as an instructor,
teacher, adviser and guide, and how this has developed to include how
to help people change their behaviour concerning the food they eat.
The dietitian, therefore, needs a range of skills, not least the ability to
use counselling skills appropriately. The reader will gain an understanding of how the different methods relate to issues of control between
dietitian and patient, of the different approaches to counselling and
the importance of maintaining boundaries concerning time and confidentiality as well as a feel for what it means to use a counselling
approach when working with a patient. Chapter 2 helps the reader
consider her patients' concerns in a structured way and in so doing
develop her capacity to empathise. As explained in Chapter 3, empathy
is one of the core conditions which, when demonstrated effectively,
is the basis for the helping relationship with the patient. Chapter 4
introduces the reader to models of the helping process and the process
of change. These provide the dietitian with frameworks to draw upon
when working with patients.

*The following questions are designed to aid the reader's reflection and
promote discussion.*

- How would you describe your personal philosophy about helping others?
- In what circumstances might you use a counselling approach?
- How would you establish boundaries for time and confidentiality? What exactly would you say?
- How would you describe, in a concise, structured way, a patient you have recently seen?
- What do the *core conditions* mean to you?
- How would you use *the helping process* and the *phases of change* to help you in an interview?

Part 2   The skills

Chapter 5 introduces the skill of active listening and aims to increase the reader's awareness of both her own and her patients' non-verbal communication. It describes how barriers make it difficult to listen and how discrepancies between verbal and non-verbal communication can lead to confusion and misunderstanding. Chapter 6 introduces the reader to different categories of verbal responses and their associated risks of creating a barrier between dietitian and patient. The meaning we attach to words gives our language the power to help or hinder the helping relationship. The way we respond reflects our attitude and purpose. The reader is introduced to the skill of reflective responding which enables her to demonstrate to her patients the core conditions she is able to offer. Chapter 7 shows how reflective responding is used to make helpful interventions which can further someone in their process of changing their behaviour. The art of skilful questioning is explored through ways to help someone change to a clearer and more realistic way of thinking. This chapter demonstrates how to apply these skills in a person-centred manner.

The following questions are designed to aid the reader's reflection and promote discussion.

- How could you use your observations to build rapport in an interview setting?
- What do you consider to be barriers to communication between dietitian and patient?
- What examples have you observed of discrepancies between verbal and non-verbal communication? How have these affected your communication?
- Which categories of verbal response are you most (and least) familiar with using?

- How have you applied (how do you intend to apply) your knowledge of the skills described in Part 2.
- What has been your experience of using (and receiving) active listening and reflective responding?
- What is your attitude towards (and thoughts about) making some of the helpful interventions described in Chapter 7?

Part 3   The patient interview

Chapter 8 introduces the reader to a framework for the patient interview and the reader is shown how to apply her skills in the different stages. The next four chapters concern the needs of particular groups of patients. Chapter 9 is concerned with loss and bereavement, Chapter 10 with parents and children, Chapter 11 with communicating across cultural boundaries and Chapter 12 is about working with patients who have difficulties with their physical and mental health. Each chapter highlights the points to consider when working with patients who have these concerns. Chapter 13 illustrates ways in which the counselling approach and the skills described throughout the book can be put into dietetic practice.

The following questions are designed to aid the reader's reflection and promote discussion.

- How do you think you could use the interview framework?
- What do you consider to be the similarities between the process of change and the process of adjusting to bereavement?
- What support might you need to work with patients who are bereaved or come from a different cultural background?
- What changes, if any, would you like to happen that would make your work with (i) parents and children and (ii) patients with physical needs, more fulfilling?
- How would you recognise if a patient was depressed or anxious to the extent that they need professional help?
- How might you use your counselling skills to help a patient who unexpectedly told you about their bizarre eating behaviour?

Part 4   Areas for personal development

Chapter 14 introduces the reader to the skills of communicating assertively and relates this to some of the difficult situations which can occur between colleagues as well as with patients. Handling such situations also requires skills of active listening, reflective responding and effective confrontation. The reader will have broadened her understanding of how these skills can be applied. Using a counselling approach when working with others, both as a colleague and as a helping professional, requires that we have support. Chapter 15 shows how the reader can give and receive support in a purposeful way.

The following questions are designed to aid the reader's reflection and promote discussion.

- When, with whom and in what situations do you want to communicate more assertively?
- How do you know when you are feeling too stressed – what are your thoughts, feelings and behaviour?
- How do you manage your stress? What new ways to unwind are you planning to implement?
- How would you explain to someone else the connections between stress, assertive communication, self-esteem and your ability to use counselling skills?
- When someone is heard, acknowledged and accepted they are more motivated to attempt making changes. Do you agree with this statement? How would you explain the process implied in the statement and what skills would you practise to enable it to happen?
- What changes (if any) are you planning to make in your dietetic practice that would ensure your greater safety and well-being?
- How could you get more support for yourself?

Appendix 1

Further Reading

Of the many books available the following are a selection of text books, self-help books, personal accounts and novels to enhance the reader's knowledge on some of the subjects raised in this book. I have added an explanatory note in brackets where the title does not obviously convey the content.

Bereavement

Helen, M. (2002) *Coping with Suicide*. Sheldon Press, London.

Hill, S. (1977) *In the Springtime of the Year*. Penguin, London. (A novel describing a woman coming to terms with a painful bereavement.)

Kelley, P. (1997) *Companion to Grief*. Piatkus Ltd, London.

Kon, A. (2002) *How to Survive Bereavement*. Hodder & Stoughton, London.

Kubler-Ross, E. & Kessler, D. (2005) *On Grief and Grieving*. Simon & Shuster UK Ltd., London.

Communication skills

Alberti, R.E. & Emmons, M.L. (2001) *Your Perfect Right*. Impact, Dublin. (A classic book on assertiveness.)

Back, K., Back, K. & Bates, T. (2005) *Assertiveness at Work – A Practical Guide to Handling Awkward Situations*. McGraw-Hill, London.

Bandler, R. & Grinder, J. (1999) *Frogs into Princes: Neuro Linguistic Programming*. Real People Press, Moab, USA. (A classic book on neuro-linguistic programming.)

Bolton, R. (1986) *People Skills*. Prentice Hall, Sydney.

Dickson, A. (1982) *A Woman in Your Own Right*. Quartet Books, London. (A classic book on assertiveness.)

Dickson, A. (2004) *Difficult Conversations – What to Say in Tricky Situations Without Ruining the Relationship*. Piatkus Ltd, London.

Dryden, W. & Constantinou, D. (2004) *Assertiveness Step by Step*. Sheldon Press, London.

Fisher, R., Ury, W. & Patton, B. (2003) *Getting to Yes*. Random House Business Books, London. (On negotiation skills.)

Hare, B. (1996) *Be Assertive – the Positive Way to Communicate Effectively*. Vermilion, London.

Lindenfield, G. (2001) *Assert Yourself*. Harper Collins, London.

O'Connor, J. & Seymour, J. (2003) *Introducing Neuro Linguistic Programming*. Harper Collins, London.

Quilliam, S. (2004) *Body Language*. Carlton Books, London.

Stewart, I. & Joines, V. (1987) *TA Today – A New Introduction to Transactional Analysis*. Lifespace Publishing, Nottingham. (A framework for understanding interactions and communications in relationships.)

Williams, D. (1997) *Communication Skills in Practice – A Practical Guide for Health Professionals*. Jessica Kingsley Publishers, London. (Includes useful sections on working in a multidisciplinary team and giving presentations.)

Counselling

Burnard, P. (1999) *Counselling Skills for Health Professionals*. Chapman & Hall, London.

Ellin, J. (1994) *Listening Helpfully – How to Develop Your Counselling Skills*. Souvenir Press, London.

Heron, J. (2001) *Helping the Client*, 5th edn. Sage Publications, London.

Houston, G. (1995) *Supervision and Counselling*, 2nd edn (rev.) The Rochester Foundation, London.

Mearns, D. & Thorne, B. (1999) *Person Centred Counselling in Action*, 2nd edn. Sage Publications, London.

Miller, W.M. & Rollnick, S. (2002) *Preparing People to Change Addictive Behaviour*. Guilford Press, New York. (On motivational interviewing.)

Pratt, J. (1994) *Counselling Skills for Professional Helpers*. Central Book Publishing Ltd, London.

Rollnick, S., Mason, P. & Butler, C. (1999) *Health Behaviour Change – a Guide for Practitioners*. Churchill Livingstone, Edinburgh.

Sanders, P. (2002) *First Steps in Counselling*, 3rd edn. PCCS Books, Manchester.

Tolan, J. (2003) *Skills in Person Centred Counselling and Psychotherapy*. Sage Publications, London.

Eating disorders

Gilbert, S. (2005) *Counselling for Eating Disorders*, 2nd edn. Sage Publications. (Using CBT as a means to help patients.)

Lemma-Wright, A. (1994) *Starving to Live – the Paradox of Anorexia Nervosa*. Central Book Publishing Ltd, London.

Orbach, S. (2005) *Hunger Strike*. Karnac Books, London. (An account of the social and cultural phenomena underlying eating disorders.)

Orbach, S. (2006) *Fat is a Feminist Issue*, 3rd edn. Arrow Books, London. (Eating disorders seen as a solution to a social and cultural problem.)

Mental illness

Axline, V. (1964) *Dibs in Search of Self*. Penguin, London. (A moving account of a child responding to therapy.)

Haddon, M. (2004) *The Curious Incident of the Dog in the Night-time*. Vintage, London. (A readable book showing insight into the mind of an autistic boy.)

McMahon, G. (2005) *No More Anxiety – Be Your Own Anxiety Coach*. H. Karnac (Books) Ltd, London. (Uses cognitive-behavioural therapy (CBT) skills and techniques.)

Rowe, D. (2003) *Depression – The Way out of Prison*. Routledge, London.

Trickett, S. (1996) *Coping with Anxiety and Depression*. Sheldon Press, London.

Personal development

Butler, G. & Hope, T. (1995) *Manage Your Mind*. Oxford University Press, Oxford. (A practical guide including a chapter on CBT.)

Field, L. (2001) *Creating Self Esteem*. Vermilion, London. (A practical guide.)

Gawain, S. (1995) *Creative Visualisation*. New World Library, USA. (Represented by Airlift Book Co., Enfield.) (A guide to developing creativity.)

Miller, A. (1995) *The Drama of Being a Child*. Virago Press, London.

Scott Peck, M. (2003) *The Road Less Travelled*. Rider & Co., distributed by Wisdom Books, Ilford. (A journey of self-realisation.)

Winnicott, D.W. (1991) *The Child, the Family and the Outside World*. Penguin, London.

Stress management

Balfour, S. (2002) *Release Your Stress*. Hodder & Stoughton, London.

Cartwright, S. & Cooper, C. (1994) *No Hassle – Taking the Stress Out of Work*. Century Ltd, London.

Greener, M. (2002) *The Which? Guide to Managing Stress*. Which? Ltd, London.

Appendix 2

Useful Addresses

The contact details of some organisations may have changed since the publication of this book. Readers are recommended to check details before passing on information to patients and colleagues.

Professional organisations

British Association for Counselling and Psychotherapy (BACP)
BACP House
35–37 Albert Street
Rugby
Warwickshire CV21 2SG
Tel: 0870 443 5252
Fax: 0870 443 5161
Email: bacp@bacp.co.uk
Website: www.bacp.co.uk

(Provides a directory of counsellors and psychotherapists and information on counselling training.)

British Dietetic Association
148/9 Great Charles Street
Birmingham B3 3HT
Tel: 0121 200 8081
Email: info@bda.uk.com
Website: www.bda.uk.com

United Kingdom Council for
Psychotherapy (UKCP)
2nd Floor
Edward House
2 Wakley Street
London EC1V 7LT
Tel: 0207 014 9955
Fax: 0207 014 9977
Email: info@psychotherapy.org.uk
Website: www.ukcp.org.uk

Some organisations related to concerns mentioned in this book

Many of these organisations have local branches and regional centres; some provide information and training for professionals; some provide a list of practitioners for which there may be a small charge.

Bereavement and terminal illness

Cruse
Cruse House
126 Sheen Road
Richmond
Surrey TW9 1UR
Tel: 020 8939 9530
Helpline: 0870 167 1677
Young person's freephone helpline:
0808 808 1677
Email: info@crusebereavementcare.
org.uk
Website:
www.crusebereavementcare.org.uk

Foundation for the Study of Infant
Deaths (FSID)
Artillery House
11–19 Artillery Row
London SW1P 1RT
Helpline: 020 7233 2090
General: 020 7222 8001
Email: fsid@sids.org.uk
Website: www.sids.org.uk/fsid/

SANDS – Stillbirth & Neonatal
Death Society
28 Portland Place
London W1N 4DE
Tel (helpline): 020 7436 5881
Tel (admin): 020 7436 7940
Website: uk-sands.org

The Compassionate Friends
53 North Street
Bristol BS3 1EN
Tel: 0117 953 9639
Website: www.tcf.org.uk

The Hospice Information Service
Hospice House
34–44 Britannia Street
London WC1X 9JG
Tel: 0870 903 3903

Child and family support

Action for Sick Children
Midlands Office
No 3 Abbey Business Centre
Keats Lane
Earl Shilton
Leicestershire LE9 7DQ
Tel: 01455 845 600
Website:
www.actionforsickchildren.org

Carers UK
20–25 Glasshouse Yard
London EC1A 4JT
Tel: 020 7490 8818
Email: info@ukcarers.org
Website: www.carersonline.org.uk

ChildLine
Studd Street
London N1 0QW
Helpline: 0800 1111
Textphone: 0800 400 222
Tel: 020 7239 1000
Email: info@childline.org.uk
Website: www.childline.org.uk

Gingerbread (for one parent families)
307 Borough High Street
London SE1 1JH
Tel: 020 7403 9500
Email: office@gingerbread.org.uk
Website: www.gingerbread.org.uk

Hyperactive Children's Support Group
71 Whyke Lane
Chichester
West Sussex PO19 7PD
Tel: 01243 539966
Email: hyperactive@hacsg.org.uk
Website: www.hacsg.org.uk

Kidscape
2 Grosvenor Gardens
London SW1W 0DH
Tel: 020 7730 3300
Fax: 020 7730 7081
Helpline: 08451 205 204
Email: info@kidscape.org.uk
Website: www.kidscape.org.uk

National Childbirth Trust
Alexandra House
Oldham Terrace
London W3 6NH
Enquiry line: 0870 444 8707
Tel: 0870 770 3236
Email: enquiries@nct.org.uk
Website: www.nct.org.uk

Parentline Plus
Unit 520 Highgate Studios
53–79 Highgate Road
London NW5 1TL
Tel: 0808 800 2222
Textphone: 0800 783 6783
Email: headoffice@parentlineplus.org.uk
Website: www.parentlineplus.org.uk

Seniorline
Freephone: 0808 8006565
Tel: 020 7278 1114
Email: info@helptheaged.org.uk
Website: www.helptheaged.org.uk

Counselling skills training

Information is available from the British Association for Counselling and Psychotherapy. For contact details see Professional organisations. Courses are also run by many local colleges.

Mental health

Depression Alliance
35 Westminster Bridge Road
London SE1 7JB
Tel: 020 7633 0557
Email: information@
depressionalliance.org
Website:
www.depressionalliance.org

Manic Depression Fellowship
21 St George's Road
London SE1 6ES
Tel: 020 7793 2600
Email: mdf@mdf.org.uk
Website: www.mdf.org.uk

MENCAP (for learning disabilities)
123 Golden Lane
London EC1Y 0RT
Tel: 020 7454 0454
Fax: 0207 608 3254
Email: information@mencap.org.uk
Website: www.mencap.org.uk

MIND
15–19 Broadway
London E15 4BQ
Information line: mindinfoline 0845
766 0163
Tel: 020 8519 2122
Fax: 020 8522 1725
Email: contact@mind.org
Website: www.mind.org.uk

National Phobics Society
Zion Community Resource Centre
339 Stretford Road
Hulme
Manchester M15 4ZY
Helpline: 0870 122 2325
Email: info@phobics-society.org.uk
Website:
www.phobics-society.org.uk

Rethink
30 Tabernacle Street
London EC2A 4DD
Frontline: 0845 456 0455
Advice line: 020 8974 6814
Email: info@rethink.org
Website: www.rethink.org

Samaritans
The Upper Mill
Kingston Road
Ewell
Surrey KT17 2AF
Helpline: 08457 909090
Tel: 020 8394 8300
Email: jo@samaritans.org
Website: www.samaritans.org.uk

SANE
1st Floor
Cityside House
40 Adler Street
London E1 1EE
Saneline: 0845 767 8000
Email: sanelineadmin@sane.org
Website: www.sane.org.uk

Seasonal Affective Disorder
Association
PO Box 989
Steyning
West Sussex BN44 3HG
Website: www.sada.org.uk

Triumph Over Phobia
PO Box 1831
Bath BA2 4YW
Tel: 01225 330 353
Email: triumphoverphobia
@compuserve.com
Website:
www.triumphoverphobia.com

Physical health and physical needs

Age Concern
Astral House
1268 London Road
London SW16 4ER
Helpline: 0800 00 99 66
Website: www.ageconcern.org.uk

DiabetesUK
Macleod House
10 Parkway
London NW1 7AA
Tel: 020 7424 1000
Fax: 020 7424 1001
Careline: 0845 120 2960
Email: info@diabetes.org.uk
Website: www.diabetesuk.net

Disabled Living Foundation
380–384 Harrow Road
London W9 2HU
Helpline: 0845 130 9177
Textphone: 0870 603 9176
Fax: 020 7266 2922
Email: dlfinfo@dlf.org.uk
Website: www.dlf.org.uk

H.E.A.R.T.UK
7 North Road
Maidenhead
Berkshire SL6 1LP
Tel: 01628 628 638
Email: ask@heartuk.org.uk
Website: www.heartuk.org.uk

Macmillan Cancer Relief
89 Albert Embankment
London SE1 7UQ
Tel: 0808 808 2020
Email: cancerline@macmillan.org
Website: www.macmillan.org.uk

National AIDS Helpline
1st Floor Cavern Court
8 Matthew Street
Liverpool L2 6RE
Tel: 0151 227 4150
Fax: 0151 227 4019
Helpline: 0800 56 7123

Pain Concern (for help with chronic pain)
PO Box 13256
Haddington EH41 4YD
Tel: 01620 822 572
Fax: 01620 829 138
Email: info@painconcern.org.uk
Website: www.painconcern.org.uk

Stroke Information Service
The Stroke Association
240 City Road
London EC1V 2PR
Stroke helpline: 0845 3033 100
Email: info@stroke.org.uk
Website: www.stroke.org.uk

Relationships

A directory of counsellors and psychotherapists is available from the British Association for Counselling and Psychotherapy. For contact details see Professional organisations.

Relate
Herbert Gray College
Little Church Street
Rugby
Warwickshire CV21 3AP
Tel: 0845 456 1310
Email: enquiries@relate.org
Website: www.relate.org.uk

Substance dependency and misuse

Al-Anon Family Groups
61 Dover Street
London SE1 4YF
Tel: 020 7403 0888
Website: www.al-anonuk.org.uk

Alcohol Concern
Waterbridge House
32–36 Loman Street
London SE1 0EE
Tel: 020 7928 7377
Email:
contact @alcoholconcern.org.uk
Website:
www.alcoholconcern.org.uk

Eating Disorders Association
103 Prince of Wales Road
Norwich NR1 1JW
Adult helpline: 0845 634 1414
Youthline: 0845 634 7650
Email: info@edauk.com
Website: www.edauk.com

FRANK (The National Drugs
Helpline)
Tel: 0800 77 66 00 (24 hours a day)
Textphone: 0800 917 8765
Email: frank@talktofrank.com
Website: http://talktofrank.com

Quitline
Ground Floor
211 Old Street
London EC1V 9NR
Advice line: 0800 002 200
Tel: 020 7251 1551
Email: info@quit.org.uk
For smokers:
stopsmoking@quit.org.uk
Website: www.quit.org.uk

Women's Therapy Centre
10 Manor Gardens
London N7 6JS
Tel: 020 7263 7860
Fax: 020 7281 7879
Email (general enquiries, including
education & training):
info@womenstherapycentre.co.uk
Psychotherapy enquiries:
appointments@
womenstherapycentre.co.uk
Website:
www.womenstherapycentre.co.uk

Well-being and stress management

Aromatherapy Organisations
Council
PO Box 6522
Desborough
Kettering
Northants NN14 2YX
Tel/fax: 0870 774 3477
Email: info@aromatherapy-
regulation.org.uk
Website: www.aocuk.net

British Acupuncture Council
63 Jeddo Road
London W12 9HQ
Tel: 020 8735 0400
Fax: 020 8735 0404
Website: www.acupuncture.org.uk

British Homeopathic Association
Hahnemann House
29 Park Street West
Luton LU1 3BE
Tel: 0870 444 3950
Fax: 0870 444 3960
Website: www.trusthomeopathy.org

British Massage Therapy Council
17 Rymers Lane
Oxford OX4 3JU
Tel/fax: 01865 774 123
Email: info@bmtc.co.uk

British School of Osteopathy
275 Borough High Street
London SE1 1JE
Tel (clinic): 020 7930 9254
Tel (enquiries): 020 7407 0222
Website: www.bso.ac.uk

British Wheel of Yoga
25 Jermyn Street
Sleaford
Lincolnshire NG34 7RU
Tel: 01529 306851
Fax: 01529 303233
Website: www.bwy.org.uk

Shiatsu Society of the United
Kingdom
Suite D Barber House
Storey's Bar Road
Fengate
Peterborough PE1 5YS
Tel: 01733 758 341
Website: www.shiatsu.org.uk

Society of Teachers of the Alexander
Technique
1st Floor, Linton House
39-51 Highgate Road
London NW5 1RS
Tel: 0845 230 7828
Fax: 020 7482 5435
Email: office@stat.org.co.uk
Website: www.stat.org.uk

Suzy Lamplugh Trust (leading
charity on personal safety)
National Centre for Personal Safety
Hampton House
20 Albert Embankment
London SE1 7TJ
Tel: 020 7091 0014
Fax: 020 7091 0015
Email: info@suzylamplugh.org.uk
Website: www.suzylamplugh.org.uk

Working with minority groups

Nafsiyat (provides psychotherapy for clients from diverse backgrounds).
Top Floor
262 Holloway Road
London N7 6NE
Tel: 020 7686 8666
Fax: 020 7686 8667
Email: admin@nafsiyat.org.uk
Website: www.nafsiyat.org.uk

Index